Praise f

Seed, Stem, Bloom: Lessons From My F   *r*
by Mary Robinson

"Mary is someone who allows herself to be completely and utterly transformed by the events of her life. In faith, perspective, humility, and in relationship with herself and all around her, she is someone who models potent resilience. Resilience often doesn't feel good or pretty, but it's the engine of transformation. Mary's embodiment of this process is honest, authentic, and hopeful."

- Katie Benway, Psychic, Medium,
Certified Life Coach at Intrepid Eleven, LLC, and author of
Ignite Your Intrepid Soul: A courageous home for your human heart

––––––––––

"Mary encompasses the true spirit of SURVIVOR. During her journey with CANcer, she always displayed an attitude of gratitude. Mary always wore a face of hope when we would see her. Mary's bubbly personality, and beautiful smile, gave those around her a sense of faith, hope, and love. Mary's unwavering perseverance offers hope that can conquer any and all obstacles. In her story, you have the opportunity to experience both her authenticity and her vulnerability. Her documented journey will give others the courage to tell their story, too."

- Methodist Estabrook Cancer Center Inner Beauty friends

––––––––––

"Mary went through treatment of leukemia twice and received hematopoietic stem cell transplantation when leukemia returned after initial treatment. Mary maintained contagious optimism through good times and bad. In this book, Mary describes how going through leukemia treatment transformed her life and led to monumental personal growth. Her powerful story is bound to uplift and inspire people and families dealing with cancer or any other crisis! A must-read for anyone looking for hope and inspiration!"

- Dr. Vijaya Raj Bhatt, Medical Director,
Leukemia Program, Fred & Pamela Buffett Cancer Center

––––––––––

"The best part of my job is getting to appreciate life through the perspective of my patients. Mary's view of life is something we can all benefit from appreciating. I am a better doctor because I know her."

~ Tim Huyck, MD, Oncologist at Nebraska Cancer Specialists

_____

"This book illustrates the strength of the human spirit. Mary is a truth-teller. Her story provides inspiration and encouragement for anyone facing a major health crisis... It can also offer guidance for someone at a crossroads in their life. She is living proof that this transitional time can be used to find and follow our inner voice, to tap into our spiritual strength, and to help us find our path and purpose."

~ Joyce Swanson, Educator, Therapist, and Energy Worker

_____

"While reading *Seed, Stem, Bloom*, memories came flooding forth, those days and nights of me sitting bedside with my life-long best friend. She received her leukemia diagnosis at the same time as the author. Robinson brought to life the tears, the laughter, the after-chemo illness, and the pain that one must endure healing through CANcer... Robinson's faith guides her throughout her story, showing her how to proceed, a touchstone in her hours of darkness and light. *Seed, Stem, Bloom* is a must-read for anyone considering their (stem-cell replacement therapy) treatment options. This book will help the individual and support people, families, friends, and the care system. I wish I had this in hand guiding me while I sat beside my dear friend."

~ Regina Ochoa, Medium, Transitions Counselor

_____

"Mary Robinson's approach to how she writes about CANcer seems inspired by her eternal faith in God. I felt as though I was an eyewitness to her inner world of Healing. A very sacred place."

~ Dr. Deborah R. Goldberg, Relationship Consultant,
Mediation Specialist, Certified Healing Touch Practitioner,
Advanced Clinical Hypnotherapist, Reiki Master

_____

"There are two kinds of challenges that people face. The first are the challenges that we willingly take on to expand our horizons and grow in service. The second are the challenges that are thrust upon us and make us grow despite the great difficulties that accompany them. We would never choose them for ourselves or others but after we have successfully overcome them, we are stronger and more resilient… The story of Mary's battles is compelling, and you will learn from her courage as you join her in 'joy hunting' though it all."

~ Ellen Lund, speaker, retreat leader, freelance writer

"This book is very uplifting. Its raw openness, authenticity, vulnerability, and honesty are truly inspiring."

~ Rhonda Buck, Faith Formation Director,
Student of Healing Touch

"Mary Robinson writes an honest and heartbreaking account of not only the toll cancer takes on your body but also how it affects a person mentally and spiritually. Through everything, she shows how faith and the love of family and friends can help overcome the most crippling of situations. This book will not only be inspirational for people going through the various stages of cancer, but it will also help loved ones understand what they are dealing with. Mary is able to eloquently describe what others may have difficulty expressing when going through such a battle."

~ Lisa Mottl

"Mary's unveiling life experience has not only enhanced my mindset but has deepened my faith and has changed my comprehension of God's will in each of our lives."

~ Shaela Blanchard, Owner of Blo Blow Dry Bar, Centennial, CO

"When Mary writes, she paints a picture in her reader's mind of the good, the bad, and the ugly. Mary's faith in God gave her courage and hope to fight her CANcer, and fight she did."

~ Sandy Tams

"Mary's strong faith and near-constant spiritual practice carry her through and provide comfort and encouragement that, with God on her side, she CAN do anything."

~ Susan Vastine

"Mary is a woman of faith that turned cancer into CANcer. Her book will give you a glimpse into her life as a mother, daughter, wife, teacher, and woman."

~ Laurie Taylor, MS,
Certified Healing Touch Practitioner, Reiki Master

"By sharing her personal story, Mary inspires others to move mountains just as she has. Mary reminds us to live beyond lists, embrace the love and connectedness of nature, and open oneself to various cultural healings in her fight with CANcer."

~ Elizabeth (Becky) Turner, School Psychologist

"This inspirational book is a must for those going through cancer treatment and those who love them. Mary's faith filled words reflect the positive strength of hope and reassurance in a power far beyond what we can understand, one that surpasses what we in medicine have to offer to truly heal one's mind, body, and spirit."

~ Kim Bland, DNP, APRN-NP, FNP-BC, AOCN

SEED

STEM

BLOOM

Lessons From

My Faith-led Journey

Through CANcer

MARY ROBINSON

Seed, Stem, Bloom: Lessons From My Faith-led Journey Through CANcer

Mary Robinson

©Copyright 2022

All rights reserved. No portion of this book may be reproduced, translated, stored in a retrieval system, or transmitted in any form or by any means, electronic, mechanical, photocopying, microfilming, recording, or otherwise without written permission from the publisher, except in the case of brief quotations embodied in critical articles and reviews.

Published by the Compassionate Mind Collaborative.

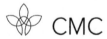 CMC

Edited by Heather Doyle Fraser

Cover design by Dino Marino

Interior layout and design by Dino Marino

Proofed by Julie Homon

ISBN: 978-1-7372006-3-5

eBook: 978-1-7372006-4-2

BE THE MATCH

If readers are interested in being on the donation list for stem cells, they can go to www.BetheMatch.org website to register. Be the Match will send a swab kit for potential donors to swab inside their mouth (cheek) and return. Potential donors will be added to the general population pool. Every life is precious and any donor could be the match for someone and save a life.

If readers are interested in donating blood, contact your local Red Cross or your community blood center to verify your eligibility and help save lives.

*To my seedlings – Brody, Holly, Colby, and Shaylee –
may you continue to blossom with each forward-moving step.*

All my love,

Mom

---

*"We are all meant to shine, as children do.
We were born to make manifest the glory of God
that is within us. It's not just in some of us; it's in everyone.
And as we let our own light shine, we unconsciously
give other people permission to do the same."*

~ Marianne Williamson

TABLE OF CONTENTS

PLANTED IN FAITH: WHERE MY STORY BEGINS

In your life's defining moments there are two choices – you either step forward in faith and power or you step backward into fear.

~ James Arthur Ray

Like most, I have had my fair share of defining moments. You know, those times in your life when something stops you in your tracks and makes you rethink your steps. It could be a simple challenge or something much more significant, like a passion project. Regardless of their intensity, these moments help redirect our lives and provide opportunities for self-discovery, encouraging growth in the pursuit of a purpose.

Once these journeys toward a purpose begin in my life, I become hyper-aware of God's signs. I look for them everywhere and follow His beacons. Why? In my case, during times of deep introspection, I am reminded of this one simple truth: God is so good! I know that I could not accomplish any of my goals without Him leading the way.

The core of this book, with its intention to share the experiences of a particularly difficult season in my life, is all about following God's signs.

During this part of my journey, I diligently shared updates with my family and friends on my CaringBridge.org page. It felt valuable and therapeutic to document everything – not only for those who cared about me, but also for myself. Looking back, it's clear that this commitment to telling my story started with my entries on that page. And so, in keeping with the origin of my self-discovery, I decided to honor CaringBridge and my journey by writing this book in letter format – letters to my friends, family, and ultimately, myself. However, I can't move forward here without acknowledging the events that led up to my cancer diagnosis.

When I was young, I always knew that I wanted to help people, but I wasn't sure in what capacity until adulthood. I remember pretending to be a teacher with my friends when I was in elementary school. We had an entire school set up in the basement: chalkboard, chalk, and small tables with chairs – it felt like a real classroom. The tiny seed I planted as a child stayed with me over the years. In 2001, I earned my bachelor's degree with a double-major in elementary education and special education (mild to moderate disabilities). After working in the field of special education for a while, I wanted to expand my studies into a specialty. So, in 2006, I began taking courses for my master's degree in special education, emphasizing in visual impairments. In 2008, I was hired on a provisional teaching certificate as a teacher of the visually impaired (TVI) while I completed the last course of my master's program. Eventually, I furthered my education even more by becoming a certified orientation and mobility specialist (COMS) in 2012. God had a plan for me, and, through it all, He remained by my side. Little did I know exactly what He had in mind for my future until my BIG project… The Sensory Courtyard, where "Seeds Sown Today Bring Blossoms Tomorrow."

As a life-long learner myself, I am always looking for new ways to help students grow. In the summer of 2011, a 'chance' encounter at a National Federation of the Blind Convention in Florida changed the direction of my life. While there, I met a family with a three-year-old boy who happened to be blind. His mother told me about his difficulties in developing skills and reaching important milestones. She feared that the educational gap was expanding to the point that he wouldn't be able to catch up to his peers. We visited for quite some time, and I found out that her son was very tactile-defensive, meaning he did not want to touch, let alone play with, toys. Oftentimes, the three-year-old sat in a corner crying when early interventionists came into their home to work on needed skills. His mother decided to quit her job and spend more time with her son in hopes of improvement through more consistent support. She decided to plant a garden in her backyard with her son, even though he demonstrated no desire to be involved. Regardless of his attitude, she made sure to expose him to the garden daily, introducing him to the assortment of plants. Over time, he began touching, picking, smelling, and tasting the vegetation. As the early interventionists continued to work with her son in their home, he began to explore! He started reaching important milestones as these tactile-defensive traits diminished, and the educational gap began shrinking to a realistic size.

After meeting with that family in Florida, a spark grew inside me. I thought, "If that mother could do this for her son from a simple garden in their backyard, then why couldn't I do something in an educational setting to help students of ALL abilities?" This dream invigorated me. I wanted to give a voice to those who could not speak for themselves, those who require alternate avenues or paths to learn, grow, and achieve.

That short visit with the boy's mother was a significant turning point in my life. Was it *really* 'chance' that led to my passion project called the Sensory Courtyard? Looking back, I know this project was greater than me – the universe guided it. Everything lined up just as it was supposed to, and I could feel that God was smiling down on my plan. This does not mean that everything was clear to me initially, though. It's easy to see these events and label them as fortunate when you look back through time, but in the moment, I needed to have all my senses on board. Most importantly, I called upon my intuitive wisdom, striving to see the path I was creating with each choice and step.

Dreaming and holding the vision of a goal in your future is a healthy, fruitful activity. If you follow and manifest one small desire, one tiny seed, you have the ability to grow the most bountiful garden. Hanging onto that vision is one of the only things that has kept me going on my journey.

It took a great deal of courage to step forward in faith and dream big when I began to work on my vision, the Sensory Courtyard. The grace of God and the substantial support from my family, colleagues, and friends made my aspiration a reality. With that being said, although the help of companions and the strength of my goal were vital, they were not the central piece to the Courtyard's success. The main contributor was my unseen diligence. I set daily intentions, weekly goals, and monthly benchmarks to keep myself on track and keep the project moving towards completion.

Ambition, faith, and confidence are critical components in moving forward with intentional thoughts. There were many days while the project was in its infant stage that I asked myself, "Is this 'pie in the sky' really coming to fruition?" When this question arose, I took a step back and, with a deep breath, realized that this dream and vision happened for a reason. The universe was working in agreement with me and this passion project. It validated my primal belief that one of the reasons God put me on Earth was to help those in need who cannot speak for themselves. My role is to be an advocate. God wants us to dream big and therefore blesses good intentions.

When I first conceptualized the vision of the Sensory Courtyard, it felt unreal, as if it was just a fantasy. How could I bring something like this to fruition? Fantasies are not transformed into reality overnight. In my case, the Sensory Courtyard took three years. And, like many plans, it had some ups and downs. Even with all its challenges, though, the signs that God placed in my path assured me that He was by my side. He orchestrated this project beautifully, and my experience helped me evolve on many levels – physically, emotionally, mentally, and spiritually.

It's important to remember that God is always with us, even when we cannot feel Him. God wrote our story even before we took our first breath. He is all-powerful, all-wondrous, all-loving, and all-knowing. God wants only the best for us. Some days may seem like a never-ending hike up a mountain with winding paths and treacherous terrain. Other days may feel like a nice, calm sunny day at the beach – having no care in the world and no worries about what is ahead. Then again, some days ignite a spark inside us, giving us a new passion for achieving what some may call 'the impossible.'

A chronicle that reminds me of this potential is centered around a French man named Jean Gravelot, nicknamed "The Great Blondin" because of his fair-colored hair. He was the first tightrope walker to cross Niagara Falls. Everyone told him, "You can't do that. You will kill yourself!" So, what did he do? He walked across Niagara Falls on the tightrope carrying a thirty-foot-long balancing pole that weighed forty pounds. Halfway through, he stopped, dropped a bottle tied to a piece of twine into a boat below, and hauled up some water to drink before finishing the mission. The Great Blondin proved everyone wrong.

As if his first accomplishment wasn't impressive enough, Gravelot wanted to step it up and walk across Niagara Falls again. His next attempt involved even more danger, as he rode a bicycle and pushed a stove in a wheelbarrow while cooking an omelet during his tightrope walk. The Great Blondin took several risks to confirm that he could do it. And after he had proved himself many times to observers, everyone's mindsets began to shift. Viewers grew to trust in him. One of his following incredible acts was to carry a man across on his back. Only now the audience was saying, "You can do it, you can do anything!"

They were all skeptical of the Great Blondin's abilities without seeing evidence of his skills. And who can blame them? It's tough to put faith in something without tangible proof. This doubt applies to our relationship with God as well. It is essential to take a blind step forward and trust that God has an incredible outcome planned for each of us. The Great Blondin had faith in himself and proved everyone wrong with that impossible walk. Like him, I needed to rely on faith and believe that my project would be successful, no matter what obstacles were placed in my path.

A friend once told me that it's important not to accept other people's belief systems about what is possible and what is not. ANYTHING is possible; we limit ourselves if we question our strength. I find myself wanting to work harder only to prove that what may seem impossible to some IS possible with determination, perseverance, and a positive mindset. I am living proof that this approach of thinking is valid. I suppose you could call it: The law of attraction.

This way of thinking was put to the test, though. As the Sensory Courtyard's necessities continued to increase, so did my student caseload and their needs. That's how it works sometimes. When you tell yourself you are ready for the hard work and ready to be of service, the universe seems to answer by throwing everything at you at once. I tried to leave behind the pressures of my aspirations when I was with my family, but there were times that I put them to the side and chose to meet deadlines or present to potential donors instead. It was a sacrifice that I was willing to make if it meant ensuring my project's completion, and I also knew late nights and early mornings wouldn't be long-term situations. Looking back, I wish I hadn't let myself become so overwhelmed.

You might be wondering why my story starts with my dream of the Sensory Courtyard. Well, to some extent, this project took over my life. I gave up a lot to make this dream happen, and in my quest, I ignored some of the signs I should have paid attention to along the way. For instance, I had faced work-related quarrels in my department nearly every day for two years leading up to my Sensory Courtyard Project. Those disputes depleted my spirit and re-exposed my subconscious feelings of inadequacy. In fact, I believe the years of destructive criticism from some of the workers in my department reminded me of the pieces of my past that hurt the most. Needless to say, their cruelty cut deep into my core.

Fortunately, God listened to my cries and helped me survive the toxic workplace. The past cannot be changed, but I *can* alter my future. My project helped me loosen the tight ropes of self-pity that choked me for so long. Despite our differences, my department tried our best to work together for the sake of the Sensory Courtyard.

The strongest ACTIONS for a woman are to
LOVE HERSELF, BE HERSELF, and SHINE
amongst those who never believed she could.

~ Unknown

Let's be honest, we live in an imperfect world that does not cater to individual circumstances. It is our duty to make the best decisions we can, with our needs in mind, as we move through fluctuating seasons of our lives. Our planet is constantly changing, and we have the freedom to make the most out of whatever is placed in our path. Attitude plays a vital role in this process of evolution. My parents' values have shaped much of my attitude about what I can achieve and what challenges I can face.

Consequently, I place high standards on myself and strive towards perfection in anything I set my mind to accomplish. Occasionally, I take this to the extreme. I'm generally sensitive to perceived faults addressed by others, and sadly, I'm also my own worst critic. I find myself playing the role of a people-pleaser and peacemaker, often apologizing and striving for harmony, wanting everyone to get along. Frequently, those around me end up happy and content, while I am internally dissatisfied from not getting my wants or needs met. Depending on how I choose to use my energy in given situations, this dissatisfaction can develop into anger and resentment.

I often find myself replaying scenarios in my mind on what I could have done differently to improve the outcome. I didn't necessarily notice these toxic reflections until I was older and identified the constant doubt as a learned habit. Perhaps, this personality trait morphed into existence from life experiences. Maybe it was already written as my life plan and was something that I needed to overcome for my soul to evolve.

Life is a balance of holding on and letting go.

~ Rumi

As the days turned into years, construction continued on the Sensory Courtyard. I had also been working behind the scenes, and the combination of my presentations and grant applications raised over one-hundred eighty thousand dollars. I put my heart and soul into this dream, and it showed. We were planning to have an open house in August 2014. Completion of the Sensory Courtyard was near.

It was currently the end of the 2013-2014 school year, and I was beyond ready for summer break. I was irritable and worn out. It had been a very hectic year keeping up with student needs, managing the construction of the Sensory Courtyard, and fitting in quality time with family. Little did I know that my aspirations would take a dramatic detour if I wanted to be alive when they were finished. The sudden diagnosis of acute myeloid leukemia was utterly heartbreaking and unexpected. Fortunately, my school district was incredibly supportive, and they put the grand opening on hold until I returned to work the following year.

As anyone could guess, this gave me much time to meditate and reflect on my life choices and inner strength. I prayed for peace, understanding, and wisdom. I also prayed for courage to have the ultimate trust in God to get me through this. I told myself that I was not a victim of cancer. After all, no matter what happens in the end, we are always victors because of the blood of Jesus. I knew Heaven would be waiting if my time was done on Earth. Psalm 34:17-18 states, "The righteous cry out, and the LORD hears them; he delivers them from all their troubles. The LORD is close to the brokenhearted and saves those who are crushed in spirit."

I had to rely on my faith to get me through this. In my life, at every difficult moment, at every place where I need to endure, I did so with Christ. In the Bible, Philippians 4:13 states: "I can do all things through Christ who strengthens me." Sometimes this scripture is difficult to remember, especially when life's trials and tribulations are at their heaviest, but its message triumphs all else.

Throughout my CANcer journey, I've discovered the importance of 'being in the moment' and not allowing distress about the past to consume me – what's done is done, and there is nothing I can do to change it. Over the years, I have developed strategies to deal with worry and self-criticism. One of those strategies is to *release* the concern. After all, being anxious about problems doesn't solve them; it simply directs all your energy into a negative state. You may be wondering exactly how I release the worry. It's really simple (although not always easy): I give all my worries to Jesus. Each moment, each day, I do my best to release these everyday problems and stressors. And, when I sense the worries creeping back, I remind myself to give them to Jesus again and again – my Savior and comforter – my Redeemer. Also, I put forth my best effort not to overly worry about what the future holds because it can change in an instant. My destiny is dependent on the choices I make right now. Isn't that wonderful to know? Stay attentive and make wise decisions.

Life is ironic. It takes sadness to know happiness,
noise to appreciate silence, and absence to value presence.

~ Unknown

During extended stays in the hospital in my CANcer journey, I listened to an upbeat Christian radio station twenty-four hours a day. These songs, along with bible verses and inspirational quotes, were my anchor in a time when I was losing sight of myself. That's why I chose to begin and end each main story with a fragment of encouragement. My deep hope is that this book – which started as letters and messages to my family and friends – brings comfort and offers guidance to others going through similar life struggles. Perhaps the valuable lessons I learned along the way will spark life in another soul.

May God bless you on your journey.

 Isaiah 46:4 ~ Even to your old age and gray hairs I am he, I am he who will sustain you. I have made you and I will carry you; I will sustain you and I will rescue you.

ONE

BALANCE IN THE SHIFTING SAND

There are times in your life when you question everything. These defining moments can be places of growth or they can be places where you feel you just might wither and die. No one can tell at the beginning of each stage how things will turn out or their significance. During these times, all you are left with is your faith and trust in God. I've had more than a few defining moments in my life, and I've come to realize that every pivotal occurrence enhances my perspective. My CANcer journey is one of the many consequential events that shifted my direction and this is my story.

ACCEPTING WHAT IS

Most of the important things in the world have been
accomplished by people who have kept on trying
when there seemed to be no hope at all.

~ Dale Carnegie

Life is nowhere near simple. The human body and mind are, at times, complicated beyond comprehension. This intricate mass of flesh and bones could only be molded by the hands of God; nothing else is capable of creating such sophisticated beauty. He gave us the blank canvas of our bodies – and with His chosen brushstrokes of hardship or prosperity, helped us develop a magnificent painting of our identity. Life's struggles are merely additions to our rich canvas.

In August of 2014, I knew something was wrong with me and I was scared. I had spent the past three years engrossed in my career passion project, the Sensory Courtyard, a magical enclosed space which aids in the progression of developmental milestones for those of all abilities. As a teacher of the visually impaired, I wanted to give this gift to the children I worked with and to the community. It was so special and had the potential to help so many. As I worked, though, especially in the months leading up to the opening, I had felt tired and I had noticed changes in my body that didn't seem normal. I am the type of person who keeps commitments and pushes through difficult situations. I am the person who never quits! I knew something was wrong with me, though, and I needed to be strong enough to find out what it was.

On August 4, I went to my family doctor. I hadn't been feeling well for several months. I knew I was worn out by the end of 2014 school year, but I blamed it all on running around from place to place, mommy duties, and just life in general. I mean, what could possibly be wrong with me? I was thirty-eight years old and felt like I took pretty good care of myself. I tried to exercise regularly, eat the right foods, and most importantly, stay active. But did I push myself too far?

About three months prior to this appointment, I was noticing little sores inside my right nostril. I would use a Q-Tip to put Neosporin on the area; it would go away for a little while, then return. I blamed it on the dry air, even though this was something that normally didn't happen to me.

During the course of the summer, I noticed that when I went on brisk walks, over-exerted myself, or ascended stairs, I would get unusually out of breath. When I completed a task, I felt tired but continued to go about my day as usual. After all, I had four kids to take care of, house duties, and project goals. I didn't have time to think about how I was really feeling. Maybe it was a little bit of denial, and certainly, there was some unspoken fear. I'm not sure why it took so long for me to really check things out. Maybe it was all in God's precious timing. I'd like to go with that for my answer. There is no reason for me to feel guilt or shame for how I handled it all.

By mid-June, I noticed a large amount of blood spewed in the sink after I flossed. My gums were very sore and a little swollen. I mentioned it to my husband, Tim, because it was alarming to me. I floss daily and have never seen so much blood from flossing. In fact, normally I didn't bleed at all. I said, "Well, we have dentist appointments in a couple of weeks. I'll ask the dentist about it if my gums are still bleeding by then. Maybe I just flossed too hard."

June 30, we all had our six-month routine dental check-up. I talked to the dentist about what I had been experiencing. I was still flossing but being more careful. He looked at my records and noticed that months prior, my gums hadn't bled at all but that day, I had thirty-eight gum bleeds when he examined me. I asked about gum disease, gingivitis... any rhyme or reason for this to be happening. I agreed to call his office in a week to see if I needed to go to a gum specialist. Neither one of us made the call to each other. I felt like my gums were getting better even though they were still bleeding a bit. So, I dismissed it.

Near the end of July, my son Colby celebrated his ninth birthday with a small group of family and friends. I had been fighting a slight sore throat, nothing too concerning, but knew I wasn't feeling quite right. A few days had passed and I was fighting a cold. At first, I didn't think too much of it, but as the days progressed, my sinuses worsened and I had fevers off and on throughout the next week. At times, I needed to change my pajamas in the middle of the night because they were drenched in sweat. I thought it was my fever breaking. I would begin my days with some energy and did the usual – laundry, picking up the house, running errands, providing summer services for some of my students, and taking care of my children's needs. By late afternoon, I was completely drained, would get low grade fevers and an achy body. It was not fun by any means. I would go to bed and lay there all evening, quarantining myself because I didn't want to risk infecting my family.

In early August, I still had symptoms of a cold, but overall, I felt okay. Most days everything began as usual, but by afternoon, I was completely drained and would often go to bed with a low-grade fever. I told Tim that I was going to make an appointment with my family doctor. On August 4, I woke up with a pain in my groin area on the right side. I felt a long strip of cysts or lymph nodes. I had some near my right arm pit too.

Luckily, I was able to see my doctor that morning. I hadn't been to my family doctor since 2011, because there was no need. When my doctor came into the room to see me, I explained some of the symptoms I'd been experiencing over the last few months and asked if he would do some blood work. He agreed and told me that they would call the next day with results from the following tests: CBC (complete blood count), along with thyroid, mono, and a cholesterol check. In the meantime, I was given antibiotics for a sinus infection. I thought, yes, I will get better just in time for the first day of school!

I received the doctor's phone call the next day, Tuesday, August 5, late in the afternoon. He said that everything came back within normal range, except I had a condition known as pancytopenia. This is when white blood cells, red blood cells, and platelets are all low. I was told that they made the first available appointment with a hematologist/oncologist from Nebraska Cancer Specialists at Estabrook Center in Omaha the following day, Wednesday, August 6, at 2:00 p.m. They called a second time and told me not to miss this appointment. When I drove to the Estabrook Center, I noticed another word in the title of that building – Methodist Estabrook Cancer Center – they had left that word out. Now I was really nervous, but took a deep breath and held my head high while walking to my appointment.

My new doctor said that I had pancytopenia, but he didn't know why. More blood work was ordered, and he scheduled a bone marrow biopsy and aspiration the following morning, Thursday, August 7, in Papillion. A bone marrow biopsy is the removal of a small amount of bone and a small amount of fluid and cells from inside the bone. I was scared and began to weep. I have always maintained to anyone going through a tough time that it is okay to cry, but that doesn't mean that I do that very often or for too long. So, in keeping with my can-do, driven attitude, I wiped away my tears and kept focusing on the future.

The morning of the bone marrow biopsy and aspiration was tough for me. I was afraid it would hurt. Yes, it was uncomfortable, but I made it through (after all, I've had four kids). A few tears rolled down my cheeks before the procedure began because of nerves, but the nurses couldn't have been nicer. I was also extremely impressed that my doctor showed up in the waiting room and visited with me for a brief moment. I felt that he truly cared about my wellbeing, even though we just met the day before.

It turns out, there was something wrong with me. Very wrong.

On August 12, I was diagnosed with acute myeloid leukemia, which is an aggressive type of leukemia and not a good one to have. Statistically, I had a forty percent chance of survival, but, thanks to my age and overall health, the odds were brought up to fifty percent. As I sat there with Tim in the doctor's office, my emotions spiraled inside of me. My doctor compassionately told me he wished that it was an easier type of leukemia to tackle and overcome. He said it could be done, but the road ahead would be full of potholes and loose gravel. I turned to my husband, and with tears in my eyes and a facade of confidence, I told him that I was in the fifty percent bracket of survival.

The next words out of my doctor's mouth hit me hard: If I didn't act quickly on chemotherapy treatments, I would only have a few months to live. So much went through my mind in that moment: What had I done wrong? How could I have prevented this? Why me? He said doctors and researchers are not sure what causes leukemia. It's just plain bad luck and I could not have prevented this from happening.

My whole life flashed in front of me and I thought of my children whom I wanted to raise and shape into respectable, hardworking, trustworthy, honest adults. I wanted to see my children graduate from high school, get married, and have children of their own... I wanted it all! I didn't want to miss out on anything with my husband or my children. And my three-year-long project, the Sensory Courtyard was almost complete. I was planning an open house for it very soon.

When I managed to take control of the disarray around me, I looked straight up to heaven and pleadfully prayed for God to have mercy on me. The only thing I could do at that moment was grab onto faith and so that's what I did. I refused to consume myself with dreadful thoughts. I wiped my tears and made a decision right then to fight with all my might to make it to the final round as the winner! In that moment, I realized just how strong I am.

I had two choices: I could fight with everything in me or I could decide to not fight. For me, this really was no choice at all. I knew I would fight with everything in me. I would fight every single day until I received the news that I was free from cancer. I knew that I would have good days and bad days, but my focus was on the future. In my mind, this diagnosis was just temporary, and it totally sucked, but I had God in the ring with me ready to take swings anytime I didn't have the strength to do so on my own. I was ready and willing. I also knew I had my family, friends, and a community who would pray for me and support me – this made all the difference.

There will always be events in life that are out of our control – good or bad. The results of the bloodwork and biopsies were not what I was hoping for, but I can still be comforted by God's powerful presence. This is just another reminder that my painting is not dull; God adds pops of color with experience and growth. I knew that by the end of this journey, my piece of art would be beyond glorious. God finds extraordinary ways to help and guide people through tough times. In the aftermath of a struggle, I knew in my heart that my relationship with God would be stronger. I told myself that I would not let fear control my situation and that I needed to look for the humor in everyday experiences – good or even not so good. This has always been my way of dealing with difficult things and I intuitively knew that I would need to lean on this way of being that I have cultivated and practiced over the years to help me on the difficult road ahead.

On Wednesday, August 13, I admitted myself into Methodist Hospital to begin the scariest process I've ever had to experience in my entire life –

this process felt extreme and hard and painful, but I made the choice to proceed so that I COULD live. I was thankful because I had a choice to live. People are killed from accidents in an instant on a daily basis. At least I *had* an option. I chose LIFE.

 Proverbs 19:21 ~ Many are the plans in the mind of a man, but it is the purpose of the Lord that will stand.

MINDSET MAKES A DIFFERENCE

*We all have an unsuspected reserve of strength inside
that emerges when life puts us to the test.*

~ Isabelle Allende

The news of cancer was a complete shock to all of my family members and friends. While my symptoms lingered and progressed over a short period of time, once I finally went to the doctor to find out what was wrong, everything happened so fast that we didn't even have time to fully process the diagnosis before treatments began. Fortunately, I had the best health care providers with a solid plan for the greatest outcome. They did a wonderful job keeping me comfortable, and with so many praying for me and providing me with inspiration to keep moving forward, I truly do feel blessed even during this challenging time.

For now, I am taking one day at a time, knowing that on August 20, my chemo treatments in the induction phase will be complete. Then, I wait seven days in isolation due to my blood count levels. After seven days, another bone marrow biopsy and aspiration will confirm the results of treatment. When the results come back, we will discuss next steps. I pray for remission, but if not, I need to do the same seven-day chemo treatment again. I refuse to worry about that right now. I am just doing my best to remain calm and stay positive. My mind is telling me that I will overcome CANcer. With God and so many friends and family by my side praying for me, this is my mantra.

Exodus 15:2 ~ The Lord is my strength and my song, and he has become my salvation. This is my God, and I will praise him, my father's God, and I will exalt him.

FINDING STRENGTH IN THE JOURNEY

Be the kind of person who dares to face life's challenges
and overcome them rather than dodging them.

~ Roy T. Bennett

It's August 18, and yesterday was not a good day. I was very nauseated from the chemo treatments and got caught up in a "feel sorry for myself" mode. If I've learned anything, it is that I need to give myself permission to take a little distance from the negative thoughts that replay through my mind while I'm alone in my hospital room. I wish I could press the 'shuffle' button and view my situation from an objective perspective. I realize that feeling sorry for myself at times is normal and most likely needed as part of this journey. This doesn't mean I am proud of feeling this way or that I gain anything from self-pity. It's not like I spend very long in that state either, but I do feel incredibly sad and angry at times. I know that this is okay and part of the process for me to move through it.

Oftentimes, I find myself looking out the hospital window, watching cars and pedestrians go by. Boy, what I wouldn't give to be able to go outside and take a deep breath of fresh air right now, while standing in the sunlight, soaking in all the blessings God has given me and my family over the years. My intuition is telling me that one day all of my senses will be reacquainted with the great outdoors.

As I continue to gaze out the window, I catch another glimpse of life walking on the sidewalk and begin to wonder what their story entails. Everyone has a story. Do they have children, work for the good of the community, are they healthy and happy? Do they find pleasure being alone or with others? My story was written before I took my first breath and has led me to this point in time. My story will continue to unfold in the months to come and I have this feeling deep within that everything is going to work for my best interest. It's an intrinsic knowing that one day I will be able to say that I fought the fight and won!

Everyone I watch walking down that street has their own elaborate agenda, taking their values, goals, and responsibilities into account for each situation. Humans make these calculated choices every day – so much that we tend to lose count. Our intuition and fact-based decisions may not always be life-changing, but choices eventually add up, and it's important to think about how each move affects the future. Individual courses of action, if given time, can shift your life in a positive, negative, or neutral direction. I am so thankful that I made the choice to call my doctor and make an appointment on August 4. I have been praying for guidance more and more while going through the many trials of CANcer and find that God has been with me every step of the way. He is there for all of us. We just need to seek Him.

 Matthew 11:28 ~ Come to me, all you who are weary and burdened, and I will give you rest.

LAUGHTER IS GOOD MEDICINE

Cheerfulness sharpens the edge and removes the rust from the mind. A joyous heart supplies oil to our inward machinery, and makes the whole of our powers work with ease and efficiency; hence it is of the utmost importance that we maintain a contented, cheerful, genial disposition.

~ James H. Aughey

Thank goodness for all the support from family and friends to help us all get through this. A close friend of mine set up a meal plan for my family to receive three meals a week while I'm in the hospital and during some of the recovery time. She did this through a free website service at www.takethemameal.com and anyone with the link can sign up to make a meal for loved ones. This really helped my family out, especially when Tim was in charge of feeding the kids on top of spending time with me at the hospital. It really eased his mind – and mine too – to know the kids were coming home from school with nutritious dinners, made with love. And here's something else I've realized, when your mind isn't worried about these little things it can focus on bigger things, like healing and attitude. I'm taking advantage of that for sure and feel so blessed that we have people supporting us.

I feel so grateful that I am able to FaceTime my children every day. It's refreshing to see them and hear how their days are going. These daily talks enable me to feel more part of their lives and bring a sense of normalcy even when nothing is actually normal. I try to put on a happy face when we talk, even if I'm not feeling so hot. My children are one of the reasons I am striving for a successful outcome. I have an attitude of gratitude and can't wait to get home to shower them with affection by giving big hugs and kisses, along with some snuggles. I don't want to miss out on anything in their lives.

Sometimes my attitude does take a hit though. Last night, I had some trouble with fevers and vomiting. When I'm faced with these difficult moments, I remind myself that I have been through so much, and I can make it through even the toughest challenges. I remember my children's voices, their laughter, and their smiles. These brief reflections of utter joy help me to persevere with the 'I can' attitude. These moments are just that – moments. They are not forever, just as my current situation is not for life. I can make it through. As I pull this thought out in those difficult times, I can come back to my foundation of strength and determination. With that power behind me, sometimes I feel like I can do anything! I even walked seven laps around the hospital this morning! I need to keep moving to stay as healthy as possible, even if it's for a short while. These thoughts motivate me.

I walk the hallways as much as possible, toting my large roll cart with chemo and other IV bags hanging from it while scanning the area to find bits of entertainment along the way. You have to be a joy hunter in this world, especially when you are facing something difficult. One day, as I was approaching the nurse's station, I noticed that one of the nurses in the hallway began to dance. With a chuckle, I said, "You are having too much fun! I wish I had some dance in my pants right now," as I slowly shuffled my feet to move forward inch by inch. The nurses all laughed and said that I would be dancing before I knew it. I love to dance, especially with my children. Dance parties are our favorite! Oh, how I long for that dance party in the future.

As I continued to walk down the hall, I saw my doctor walking towards me. He stopped and asked me if I had been exercising and moving around enough. I told him that I was an obedient patient and always listened to the doctor's orders. In fact, the nurses had a good laugh when I first arrived at the hospital, because I had brought light weights and jogging shoes to the hospital, with the intention of using them regularly. I quickly learned that I would not be running any marathons while in the hospital. There are some amusing times here and I am so thankful that I am allowing myself to see them and experience each one. After all, laughter is good medicine!

Crazy as it sounds, I am also having the most vivid and adventurous dreams lately! It's funny, I will go to sleep and find myself in my hometown, driving on the dirt roads around the beautiful cliffs with my friends. Or I will be on a wild ride in a car that is about to explode, but I make it out in the nick of time! Then, I wake up with a smile on my face. I realize that I don't have to be doing something to have adventure in my life. I need to remember to take this time to rest and be thankful for all the strength I've been given. Additionally, I have gratitude for the perspective I am able to inhabit because of my life experiences up to this point and what I choose to focus on. All of these things – even the CANcer – will only make me stronger in the end.

I'm going to head out for a peaceful walk now, making my dreams come true, one step at a time.

 Philippians 4:6-7 ~ Do not be anxious about anything, but in everything by prayer and petition, with thanksgiving, present your requests to God. And the peace of God, which transcends all understanding will guard your hearts and minds in Christ Jesus.

Small bits of Hope

I have been hospitalized for eight days now and will have completed the first phase of chemotherapy by this afternoon. This first round of chemo in the induction phase was intense, both mentally and physically. It consisted of chemo treatments twenty-four hours a day for a total of seven days. During the induction phase, I needed blood and platelet transfusions because my blood counts were running too low in some categories.

I was pleasantly surprised to see my doctor again last night, because normally he only sees me in the morning. I have been waiting very patiently to hear the result of one test that is extremely important and will affect my chemo plan. We were waiting for my chromosomal factors (cytogenetics). The only way I can explain it, is that there are good, fair, and bad cytogenetic categories, (AKA: The good, the bad and the ugly). I was in the good category and he came to my room last night just to let me know. My doctor is the best! The medical health care team has high hopes that my body will respond very positively to the chemo and we will be able to continue moving forward. I feel so blessed. God has this, I just know it!

It's the small bits of hope that matter the most right now. This news has definitely lifted my spirits. I will continue to move forward positively.

 Psalms 30:11-12 ~ You have turned my mourning into joyful dancing. You have taken away my clothes of mourning and clothed me with joy, that I might sing praises to you and not be silent. O LORD my God, I will give you thanks forever!

PRAYER SHAWL: HEALING COMFORT

Faith is to believe what you do not see;
the reward of this faith is to see what you believe.

~ Saint Augustine

What is normal? That's what I find myself asking most days. In the past, "normal" would have meant something different to me. It would have brought thoughts of consistency, predictability, and comfort. My new normal – at least my normal for now – looks different. It is characterized by uncertainty, unpredictability, and discomfort. So when something comes into my day that might relieve those feelings, I eagerly look for even a pinprick of light that might calm the chaos my body seems to be experiencing.

On August 20, my new normal brought me chills, fevers, muscle and body aches, hot flashes, and finally something else. I received a package from my daughter, Holly's piano teacher. Our family adores her. She's been teaching Holly for a number of years and thoughtfully brought me a gift. After I received it, I opened it and then set it aside not realizing the power of the miracle waiting for me. She had given me a prayer shawl – one that she had painstakingly made with a group of women from her church. It was made especially for me, as a reminder that a group of women is praying on my behalf. I was told that when people knit prayer shawls, they knit three stitches and purl three while stating the mantra, "In the Name of the Father (stitch one), in the Name of the Son (stitch two), in the Name of the Holy Ghost (stitch three)." On the number three purl stitches, the knitter states the name of the shawl recipient, in my case, Mary. The act of creating a prayer shawl like this can be profound and the shawl itself can provide great comfort to the wearer. I believe that God can and does reach out to each one of us in tangible ways. So, when I read on her card that I would feel God's loving arms holding me, and His unconditional love and healing ministering to me as I wear the prayer shawl, I didn't need much convincing.

And yet, as I was suffering through my chills and fevers, aches, and hot flashes, I forgot about the miracle package sitting next to my bed. After several hours of continued discomfort, my nurse said, "Mary, maybe you should put the shawl on." Of course, I said, "Please help me put it around my shoulders." Within a few minutes, I noticed the most amazing changes happening in my body. I was completely restored from the chills that were violently shaking my body. I have never experienced anything like this before and completely believe that God was embracing me, healing me with His love and compassion.

As the night progressed my fever returned and the chills began again. Once more, my nurse asked me if I wanted my shawl. I said yes, and within a couple of minutes, I was completely free of the chills. I am a walking testament of the power of love and prayer – not once, but twice in one day!

So, where does that leave me now? A believer for sure, but a truster, and a receiver as well. I know that God does not want me to suffer and does not want me to stay in this type of "normal" forever. I know He wants me to receive His loving mercy through the kindness and gifts – of others. So, I shall continue on with each forward-moving day that gets me one step closer to a healthy normal.

 Isaiah 41:10 ~ So do not fear, for I am with you; do not be dismayed, for I am your God. I will strengthen you and help you; I will uphold you with my righteous right hand.

THIS GIRL IS ON FIRE!

What the caterpillar calls the end of the world,
the master calls a butterfly.

~ Richard Bach

I have always thought of myself as someone who can physically handle pretty much anything that is thrown my way. And while I still stand by that statement, I had an experience last night (or rather early this morning on August 22) that took me completely by surprise. The short version of this story can be summed up in two small words: Hot flash! However, since I enjoy telling a tale and really making the most of the details, here's the rest of the story:

Last night I was extremely hot... uncomfortably hot! Remember Pebbles, the character in *The Flintstones* cartoon? A bone was used to hold her hair in a dainty bun on top of her head. Well, last night Pebbles and I could have been twinsies. I was ready to do anything to make sure nothing was touching my clammy neck – not even one strand of hair! I'm sure I looked ridiculous, but all I wanted last night was relief from the excruciating heat emanating from my own body! Obviously, all the covers were off, but I did still have my compression system on and doing its work on my calves. The compression system is great by the way! It wraps around my calves and blows air into a cloth-like material in a systematic way to help prevent blood clots. I have them on all night, every night. It feels like my calves are getting a mini-massage. Even when I feel like I am on fire, I'll take a massage!

Anyway, after some time, I finally fell asleep and awoke early in the morning, to find myself literally drenched in sweat. Yes, I am using the word literally correctly here. I was baffled because I was so wet. It was almost as if someone had poured a bucket of water on me while sleeping and I am not exaggerating one bit. My hair was still in place (saturated, but stable). I had fallen asleep with ice packs on each arm to help alleviate the rash and intense heat coming from them, so I checked to see if they were leaking – that would explain all of this water! Alas, no – they were bone dry! I immediately pushed the nurse's call button to see if there was anything we could do to help my comfort level because I was still hooked to the IV. They were all surprised that I was soaked – my entire shirt – front to back, but the good news was that my fever was gone for a short while after that. When my antibiotics were complete, my nurse unhooked me so I could shower and freshen up. My bedding was changed and she brought a new set of fashionable scrubs. Never underestimate the power of a shower, clean sheets, and clean clothes. I felt like a new woman!

I did learn that anything I bring from home to wear has to be washed separately from the rest of my family's laundry. And, it must be washed twice before drying. Good thing I'm wearing the hospital's scrubs! Now Tim just needs to wash my toxic whitey-tidies! So, here's to chemo side effects and menopause! This was definitely not one of the side effects I was expecting. And honestly, if someone had told me about it, I don't think I would have totally believed or understood the extent to which my body would sweat out all of these toxins. Sometimes it's hard to remember that our bodies want us to live and they are doing their best to keep us strong and alive.

So today, I am sitting here in awe of my body and my God – not for the first time and definitely not for the last I am sure. Thank you God, for giving me the strength to make it through these difficult times when I've needed You most. I believe each day will get better. I need to keep focusing on the future and what God has in store for me. I know God won't give me more than I can handle. And I know that my body is along for the ride to do its best to deal with all that is happening.

Honestly, before this happened to me, I hadn't given much thought to what women go through during their change of life transition. Yes, I've heard women complain a time or two that their ears were on fire or that they needed to use a sheet of paper as a fan to get some relief from the heat. This was not new information, but I was not able to fully relate since I hadn't experienced it for myself – that is until last night! Now, my eyes are open. I have a new appreciation and respect for women going through menopause. This intense experience was a reminder of my 'not so sympathetic' self, along with some chuckles when others going through hot flashes made remarks. I never really thought it was *that* bad, until it actually happened to me.

I find it intriguing that the human body knows exactly what to do to heal and keep us in the best mental state possible when we are experiencing these challenges. I believe some women struggle with this emotionally, almost as if there is shame around menopause when it is a natural process and progression into another stage of life. Yes, it is the end of one chapter, but also the beginning of another.

My body is going through a lot and if it (and God) decide that it's in my best interest to move forward, into the next segment; what's the shame in that? Absolutely nothing. Adios, sayonara, shalom, my long-time friend! Here's to new beginnings – bring 'em on!

 2 Corinthians 1:3-5 ~ All praise to God, the Father of our Lord Jesus Christ. God is our merciful Father and the source of all comfort. He comforts us in all our troubles so that we can comfort others. When they are troubled, we will be able to give them the same comfort God has given us. For the more we suffer for Christ the more God will shower us with his comfort through Christ.

ADVOCATE FOR YOURSELF

*Don't judge. You don't know what storm
I've asked her to walk through.*

~ God (Anonymous)

I feel obligated to keep things real and allow you into my story of survival. It's not only therapeutic for me, it lets you know that I am doing my best to keep a positive attitude, but sometimes things go wrong and get extremely scary. Last night was one of those very scary times for me.

It began like any other evening. The nurses administer four different kinds of antibiotics throughout the late evening (some in the daytime as well) and then I try to get some sleep. It's difficult to sleep during this time because nurses are in and out changing IV bags. It was about 11:30 p.m. and I noticed my right arm hurt badly. In fact, the pain turned into a tingling, numb feeling as it shot down to my middle and ring fingers.

I pushed the call button for a nurse because I have never experienced pain like this. When one of the nurses arrived, I told her what was going on and she asked what I would like to do. I thought in my head, "What would my infectious disease doctor do?" He is brilliant and always knows what to do when I have questions about anything. When I got here on August 13, I was still having minor complications from a tetanus shot I received on August 4, and my infectious disease doctor said to keep an ice pack on my arm for a few days.

I decided to ask the nurse for an ice pack and settled back into bed. A few minutes later, I popped up and knew something was terribly wrong. My body reacted strangely all of a sudden. I immediately pushed the call button for the nurse. When my nurse for the evening arrived, I told him that I felt really strange and had pain on the top-right side of my head. Through tears, I gently blew my nose. There was a long-stringy blood clot and pool of blood in my Kleenex. My mouth began tingling and got numb. There was a metallic taste in my mouth and I could taste blood at the back of my throat. At times it felt like there was a knot in my throat when I swallowed. It felt like I had a small bleed deep in my sinus area. My platelets were so low – they were at 7,000mcL – and that's when they normally provide another platelet transfusion. So, needless to say, I was worried that it would continue to bleed until I was given more platelets. The normal range for platelets is between 150,000 and 450,000 platelets per microliter (mcL).

My nurse turned off the IV and sat with me for a while. I was so scared. I asked for my prayer shawl and prayed to God for His mercy and love. I got my pocket-size scripture book out that my friend's mother-in-law had recently given me. I've been slowly studying scripture when I feel up to it and turned to the page that I've read multiple times: "Christ has redeemed me from the curse of the law. Therefore, I forbid any sickness or disease to come upon this body. Every disease germ and every virus that touches this body dies instantly in the name of Jesus. Every organ and every tissue of this body functions in the perfection to which God created it to function, and I forbid any malfunction in this body, in the name of Jesus." (Ga. 3:13; Rom. 8:11; Gen. 1:31; Matt. 16:19)

I feel like the above Word is where God leads me to often and that it was written for me in this time of trouble. After I had calmed down a bit, my nurse asked, "Should we try the IV again?" I was hesitant and asked how much longer it had. He said about fifteen minutes, so I agreed to try. He retubed the IV and started the pump. Within a minute or two, I began feeling all the terrible symptoms as before. I told him to stop the IV and that I refused to ever take that medication again. I said I would even sign a paper if needed.

He understood and literally threw the medicine in the trash. In the meantime, I was wondering what to do about all of my symptoms. Does a person take Benadryl or something else to stop this reaction? Nothing was given to me. I immediately wrote down every symptom that I experienced and the steps that were taken so I would not forget to tell the doctor about anything in case it was important. I also researched the medicine (Cefepime Hydrochloride Solution) that was in my IV bag when this happened. I found that there could be unusual or allergic reactions to those who are allergic to penicillin antibiotics. I happen to be allergic to penicillin. I asked the nurse if penicillin allergy was in my records and it was. I also asked if I needed a wristband that stated ALLERGY. I eventually got a band later that morning. I kept my prayer shawl wrapped around me all night and eventually fell asleep.

Around 4:30 a.m., I got up and took a shower, still not feeling right. I had the same mouth issues and could taste blood at the back of my throat. I was still scared. Around 6:00 a.m., I asked to speak to one of my doctors. I know my body, and something was not right. They were hesitant due to the early time, but I was persistent. I said, "Listen, I'm not a hypochondriac. You have been with me two nights in a row. I'm normally an easy patient, but I know my body. I am my own advocate and if I can't help myself, then who can?"

By 7:15 a.m or shortly thereafter, a physician's assistant came. She has seen me several times and knows my personality. I told her everything, pretty much reading what I had written. She said she would get the ball rolling fast for platelets to help clot blood, then give two units of red blood cells (carry oxygen throughout the body). She said this was real and scary, but assured me that I would be just fine. She told me that she was available all weekend. I was so grateful that she was my advocate to get things moving quickly. I have so much respect for my team of doctors.

I was given Benadryl along with my other meds. The transfusions began around 8:30 a.m. and just finished around 3:30 p.m. I slept the day away, but felt much better. Afterwards, I gently blew my nose and there was no trace of blood on the Kleenex. The micro-bleeding had stopped. I pray something like this doesn't happen again. Beating CANcer is enough work. I don't need this on top of it all. Thank God for being with me last night, wrapping me in his tender loving arms.

I have spent too many years worrying about what others think of me from my actions. It's about time I begin to stand up for myself. For some reason, it has always been easier for me to take charge when it comes to the needs of others, but not for myself. I guess cancer has pushed me into advocating for my needs. Everyone has to start somewhere at one point or another.

Jon Accuf states, "Don't compare your beginning to someone else's middle." Everyone has a beginning, middle and end. In the past, I would tiptoe to get my point across, not to hurt feelings. However, now that my life depends on positive forward-moving steps, action needs to be taken, and quickly. I was so proud of myself for speaking up and will keep reminding myself to do this from now on. I realize that it's difficult to break old habits, but with time and practice, I will overcome and prevail by advocating with a gentle heart. I refuse to miss out on joy any longer by keeping a closed mouth and sheepish attitude for fear of hurt feelings. After all, the only one getting hurt in these instances is me. I will speak my truth. This is my beginning to rediscover a joyful heart. And I'm tired of walking in the shadows.

 Deuteronomy 31:6 ~ Be strong and courageous. Do not be afraid or terrified because of them, for the LORD your God goes with you; he will never leave you nor forsake you.

TEMPORARILY DETACHED

Start over; my darling. Be brave enough to find the life
you want and courageous enough to chase it. Then start over
and love yourself the way you were always meant to.

~ Madalyn Beck

Tim had been out of town working since last Saturday and he just got back this afternoon. He had prior work-related commitments and didn't want to leave me for a week, but I assured him that I was in good hands here. Fortunately, we have the capability of using FaceTime so we can see each other every day (the kids have it too, so we can always be connected). It's so helpful because then I feel like we are together for a short while and I don't have to risk more germs in this critical time of my healing.

When Tim showed up in my room, I was shocked to see that he shaved his head – bald! I laughed and said, "What on earth did you do that for? You didn't need to do that for me!" He said he wanted to support me. What a thoughtful gesture.

Today, I began brushing my hair and was surprised at how much was coming out of my scalp. Apparently, Tim's act of shaving his head came just at the right time. I knew that I would lose my thick mane, but wasn't prepared for it to REALLY happen. I finally decided that I would NEVER finish gathering all the loose strands, so I put my remaining locks in a ponytail to keep them from getting all over my fashionable scrubs. I quickly made an appointment for the big shave with Inner Beauty at Methodist Estabrook Cancer Center.

Of course, I knew this moment was going to happen sooner or later. I just wasn't prepared for the uneasy feeling it presented. Don't get me wrong, I wasn't sad or depressed. It was just awkward to pull out my ponytail holder and see a big chunk of hair stuck in it without me even 'feeling' it come out. It's so strange to run my fingers through my hair and literally have a big clump of it in my hand, but not be able to feel the strands come out of my head. Every time I look in the trash recently there's a big pile of hair on top, but I'm not suffering pain from it falling out. I also wake up in the morning to find my hair all over the pillow, sheets, and scrubs. In fact, finding these locks all around me is more traumatic than to just shave it off, because the time had come for me to face the inevitable – there was nothing I could do to stop it.

Not to get too personal or to offend anyone, but as I said before, I want to keep this real. Another obstacle that I've needed to overcome was an embarrassment from my pubic hair falling out. Yes, when a person goes through chemo, they lose ALL their hair – a few are lucky enough to keep their eyebrows, but it depends on the type and dosage of chemo. I always have to urinate in what they call a 'hat.' It catches the urine so they can measure how much you are eliminating in a twenty-four-hour period throughout the day and night. Every time I go, more hair falls out and I refuse to reach in the 'hat' to remove it.

For the past four nights, I've had male nurses during the evening shift. At first, I thought, "Oh no, how am I going to get through this embarrassment that cannot be helped!" So, the first time the male nurse was going to dump my hat, I simply said, "Hey, just so you know, I am losing my pubic hair. Sorry for the mess." He chuckled and was so easy-going and untroubled by it. I was glad I said something because I didn't feel awkward around him afterward. My issue was 'matter of factly' stated and he was more than understanding. I guess I should be grateful that eventually, I will have the Brazilian wax look without the wax! I always wondered what they were like and I will find out soon enough without spending the money or going through the pain of waxing. By the way, the male nurses I've had are just as compassionate as the females. I shouldn't have been so uncertain. God is looking after me and making sure I am receiving the best care possible.

G.I. MARY JANE

Stay strong. The heartiest plants survive because they
weather the storms and never stop reaching for the light.

~ Robert Clancy

I felt so liberated when the cosmetologists from Inner Beauty came to my room and shaved my head. It was as if a weight was lifted and this was another new milestone that I had conquered. I finally had relief from all of my hair duties – no more brushing out loose strands or clearing it off my clothing and bed. Prior to my appointment, I sent the cosmetologists a current photo of me so they had an idea of what my hair looked like before. They brought five wigs of various colors, styles, and lengths. After I tried each of them on, Tim said, "I felt like I just had a date with five different women!" I added, "And with the same personality!" Our time with the cosmetologists was lighthearted and enjoyable. We had some good laughs. I loved the color of the first wig (Tim liked the length) and the style of the fourth wig. So, I chose the fourth wig, in the first wig's color. During our time together, we found out that some insurances cover a portion or entire cost of wigs for CANcer patients. My insurance pays up to five hundred for a wig and cleaning products to maintain it.

I won't be wearing a wig around the hospital or at my house (when I am allowed to return home); however, I do plan to wear it when we are out in public. In my mind, having a bald head makes me stick out. I don't want to be stared at or for people to feel sorry for me. I want them to see me, not the cancer. This wig will give me security and confidence, but I have to tell you... I am SO confident walking the halls with a mask covering my face and a shaved head right now. I feel beautiful inside and out, no matter what anyone else thinks of my appearance.

After all the excitement of trying on the wigs, I decided to go for a walk around the halls with Tim, and visit with the nurses. Tim said, "Doesn't Mary look like Sinead O'Connor?" But I said, "No way, I look like Demi Moore in the action movie G.I. Jane – except I am G.I. Mary Jane and kicking CANcers butt!"

Later on, two nurses came into my hospital room to administer an antibiotic. One of them said, "Mary, look what five of us (nurses) did for you!" Tears welled up in my eyes as I read a banner that said, "G.I. Mary Jane" and in the middle was a photo of Demi Moore from the G.I. Jane movie with the words "Failure Is Not an Option" and on the bottom was "Kickin' Cancer's Butt One Day at a Time!" My nurses are so awesome and this kind gesture meant more than they will ever know. I find myself looking at it all the time. Now when I walk the halls, the nurses say, "How's it going, G.I. Mary Jane?" It brings a heartening smile to my face as I continue onward. I AM kicking CANcer's butt! Thank God for the strength given to make it through each day.

 Proverbs 12:25 ~ Anxiety weighs down the heart of a man, but a good word cheers it up.

BREATH OF LIFE

Each breath is like a little rebirth, a renaissance that can only be celebrated if we recognize it's happening.

~ Cristen Rodgers

I have had another unexplainable occurrence. You can call it divine intervention or another miracle – either way, it was truly remarkable and gave me even more hope. On August 23, I was getting settled into bed. The lights were off, my eyes were closed, and I was exhausted from a day of receiving blood and platelets to sustain my life. I was praying to God; asking that all my organs run as they should and my heart stay strong and pump as it ought to, as He intended.

I was scared because of a slight pressure in the middle of my chest. A Christian song was playing in the background called, "Greater" by MercyMe. I have always been moved by this song. The lyrics begin with such a powerful message… "Bring your tired, and bring your shame. Bring your guilt, and bring your pain. Don't you know that's not your name? You will always be much more to me…" It was as if the song was on repeat and time stopped. The words of the song began to fade away while the instrumental portion continued. It was the strangest happening I've ever experienced – truly unexplainable, there are no words that would do justice to the feeling I had as I listened to the music. It was as if I was as light as a feather and completely at peace and in the moment.

Perhaps, I was in a meditative state and gradually, the only part of the song I heard was the beat of the music, fading in and out. All of a sudden, I felt a gentle breeze on my face; a cool breath of fresh air. I automatically breathed in ever so calmly and could feel air moving through my nostrils and into my lungs. I opened my eyes and nothing was there. I felt a sense of peace as tears slowly streamed down my cheeks and onto my pillow. I thanked God for His presence. If it wasn't God, then I know it was one of his helpers or a guardian angel. Who knows, all I do know is that it happened and my faith is stronger for it.

In the book of Matthew, Jesus says to the disciples, "Truly I tell you, if you have faith as small as a mustard seed, you can say to this mountain, 'Move from here to there,' and it will move. Nothing will be impossible for you." Now, I'm sure Jesus didn't mean that we can literally move mountains, but through Him and FAITH, we have the power to make a positive change, whatever that may be and nothing can stop it if it's holy.

Another thought came to my mind when this remarkable experience happened. I thought of the book of Genesis. It states, "Then the LORD God formed a man from the dust of the ground and breathed into his nostrils the breath of life, and the man became a living being." Yes, I'm already alive, but I'd like to think that the breath given to me was a healing breath to help my organs perform as they should. Immediately after this awareness, the pressure on my chest completely disappeared.

I will rest well tonight, knowing that the peace of God's love surrounds me and will continue to keep breathing in His healing breath of life. I trust this journey will be an amazing lesson of faith.

 Psalm 4:8 ~ In peace I will lie down and sleep; for you alone, oh Lord, make me dwell in safety.

Bone Marrow Biopsy

The day finally arrived for the bone marrow biopsy and aspiration on August 26. I have a choice of sedation this time since I'm in the hospital, but figured I have enough drugs running through me right now, so I am choosing to decline this service. If I could make it through the last bone marrow biopsy without sedation, then I'm sure I can handle it this time, even though it's not a fun experience.

They numb the pelvic bone area on my backside just enough to make it tolerable. This is the same medicine they use to numb for mole removals and it stings during the injection. The first time the site is numbed, they rub the area afterward and wait a few minutes. Then, they go in again with the numbing medicine and tap on the bone. After a few minutes, they perform the procedure. I mostly experienced a lot of pressure. It only takes about five minutes for them to get what they need once it's numb, but it seems longer. When they are finished, a bandage is put on the site. The site is tender for a few days – kind of like someone used your pelvic bone as a punching bag.

In about four days we will have the results. If I am in remission, I will go to the next phase (consolidation) in four to six weeks for more chemo. This phase may take up to six months. I need to come to the hospital every four weeks for many rounds of chemo treatments to make sure there are not any bad cells lingering. In this phase, we need to give my body time to build up healthy cells before I can undergo another round of chemo. I will also be able to go home when my doctor says my blood counts are high enough – sometime during that four to six-week block of time – to rebuild my strength and immune system. I will also be required to go in for lab work regularly to determine if blood transfusions or platelets are needed during the recovery time.

If the results show improvement, but not total remission, then I need to immediately redo the seven-day chemo that I just finished. Tim wants me to be prepared for this so my heart isn't completely crushed if the outcome is not in my favor. Every ounce of me believes I'll move to the next phase. I believe in the power of my body and the power of prayer!

Prayers have meant the world and helped me get through this phase of recovery. God hears all our prayers and cries for help. I know He has a plan for me and I can't wait to see it beautifully unfold in the months to come.

1 Peter 5:7 ~ Cast all your anxiety on him, because he cares.

DESTINED FOR SUCCESS

Seize every opportunity that life offers you, because when opportunities go, they take a long time to come back.

~ Paulo Coelho

Lately, with all of the heaviness around me, I have been looking to light-hearted comedies to bring some humor and a little fun to my days, especially since I am not doing normal things and feeling pretty isolated in my home and routine. I highly recommend the movie, "Nacho Libre" starring Jack Black. It's silly but filled with life lessons thrown in and a good-hearted twist at the end. This movie has come to my mind a lot lately. Not only do Jack Black's expressions remind me of my brother, Matt, but Jack has also always seemed to be a down-to-earth kind of guy in real life.

In a nutshell, 'Nacho' played by Jack Black, grew up in an orphanage with monks and has always been the cook. In one of the scenes, Jack is literally pouring scoops of 'slop' into bowls for the monks to eat. They begin complaining about the food and how there is no flavor or spice. One monk even makes the comment that "he has had diarrhea since Easters!" Boy, can I relate to that these days. The effects of chemo and all these antibiotics have been extreme!

So, Jack decides that maybe he's meant to do something greater than just cooking for the monks and orphans. I don't want to give anything away, but everything the main character (Jack Black) does is for the good of the children at the orphanage. They motivate him to be the best he can be and achieve his life's dreams.

We are all destined to do great things in our lifetime, even if we don't see what our path is right away. Sometimes it takes longer for us to figure out exactly what that greatness is, but when it's found, sparks fly, passion rises, and it's unstoppable! God has a plan for all of us. My plan has taken a detour for the moment, but there are signs guiding me on the right path to follow and taking me to the road of destiny again. Or maybe I'm not a detour at all. Perhaps this is all part of the path and the divine plan. I have complete hope that I am where I need to be and doing what I need to do. I must take this walk of faith, trusting that God has my plan intact for survival.

 Philippians 1:6 ~ Being confident of this, that he who began a good work in you will carry it on to completion until the day of Christ Jesus.

FAMILY TIES

Family gives you the roots to stand tall and strong.

~ Unknown

As I sit here, in the confined walls of my hospital room, I slowly drift off in a daydream that recaps some of my childhood memories with my parents and brother. With great reflection of my personal story, I feel that I come from a dedicated, hard-working family line. When the people in my family set out to confront challenging or difficult situations in life, we are dedicated to creating the best outcome possible. I was taught from a very young age to push through difficult situations, to work hard, and not take anything for granted. These morals and principles were taught to me since birth. Some say that souls choose their parents based upon the experience desired on earth. I am open to this way of thinking and also that we have the freedom to be reincarnated in order to advance our learning of love and evolve in light even further. I believe our purpose in life is centered around LOVE.

 1 Corinthians 13:13 states, "And now these three remain: faith, hope and love. But the greatest of these is love."

I have been reflecting on a conversation that my mom and I had over the phone a couple days ago. She told me that she just loves reading my posts on CaringBridge and that my dad and her did not realize my faith was so strong. They are so proud of me and thought it was beneficial for

Matt (my brother) and me to attend a parochial school for a few years in Columbus, Nebraska before moving to Chadron, Nebraska.

My mom was a teacher at the same parochial school where my brother and I attended in Columbus, so they did not have to pay tuition for us. In fact, my mom was my kindergarten teacher! I loved having my mom as my teacher, but I have to admit, I had jealous moments. I craved all of her attention. I found out quickly that I wasn't going to get very far with bad behavior. I remember the class singing, "The Ants Go Marching One by One, Hurrah, Hurrah" while rubbing two musical wooden sticks together to keep the beat. Well, I wasn't rubbing my sticks in sync with everyone else. My mom wasn't happy about this, so she sent me to the corner. I couldn't believe it! I learned my lesson quickly... Mom was a teacher of many, not just me, but I had what others didn't – her love and attention after-school hours.

When I was in the middle of fifth grade (my brother in seventh), we moved to Chadron because my dad acquired a position at Chadron State College as a professor. The family didn't want to move, but my dad had worked hard to earn a doctorate in education degree (Ed.D) and this was a great opportunity for him. I remember how sad I was to leave my best friend. This was a new chapter in our lives and a scary one for me. Would I be accepted in this new community so far away from home?

It took some time, but eventually, I made some great friends in Chadron's public school system. It was a culture shock for me at first. I had lived a sheltered life, but through the grace of God, I made it through grade school, high school, and then went onto college at Chadron State College (later on going to UNL, then UNCO). It was meant to be.

My dad was the oldest of ten and had a difficult upbringing, but that didn't hinder his success. His parents had very little money and remained that way until his parents' death. As the oldest child, high demands were put on my dad by his father and if something was not completed to his satisfaction, my dad would suffer both physical and verbal consequences. Subsequently, he made himself less visible by retreating into books. Reading and learning became a way to escape his father's destructive behavior. Reading proved to be a release from the pressures of perfectionism and unworthiness. Books allowed my dad to soar with his imagination and gain a wealth of knowledge in many subject areas. In the process, he became known as a 'jack of all trades.'

My dad left home as soon as he graduated high school and joined the Air Force, never looking back. That is until he received a call from his mother saying that his father had a stroke and it was necessary that he come home to take care of the small family business. Family needs took precedence over his dreams and aspirations for a bit because family takes care of family.

Over the years, my dad reconciled his relationship with his father, but our family didn't visit my grandparents often when I was growing up. Even so, I have fond memories of time spent with them. Time, experience, and age must have softened my paternal grandpa's heart and we rarely discussed the trials my dad had to endure while being raised.

My dad has such a tender heart and soul but doesn't display it often. I believe he is sensitive, like me, and has his own set of insecurities from the past, hidden deep within. On rare occasions, when I take a closer look at him, I detect a glimpse of sadness permeating through his soft blue eyes. I've always wondered if he still feels some of the pain that was placed upon him all those years ago, and has bottled those emotions up and thrown them out to sea, not allowing us to see the scarred child within. But they say scars build character, and my dad most definitely has that.

My dad has always been my hero. He is the most intelligent man I know, who can literally do anything in my eyes. He used to make toys for Matt and me when we were younger because we didn't have a lot of money, but we were happy and valued everything received with open arms. I can ask my dad anything and he almost always knows the answer. If he doesn't know, he will find out because that's the way he is – very knowledgeable and has never lost the desire to learn.

My mother was raised much differently than my dad. She was the middle child of two siblings and came from an upper-middle-class Christian family. Her dad was a farmer and her mom stayed at home to take care of the house until the kids were raised, later working outside the home. Living in the country gave mom many opportunities to explore nature with her siblings. Her grandparents ran a hybrid iris business. My mom worked for them in the garden to earn some extra cash and continues to have a love for flowers to this day.

My mom and I are a lot alike in personality – very social, outgoing, positive, and try to always see the good in situations. While I was growing up, mom was the glue that held our family together. Even though she is mousey in size, her heart is ginormous. Mom is the peacemaker and optimist. We have so many laughs together and a lot of fun. She is my best friend and one that I can always count on, cry with, and lean on for support.

I have always been private about my spiritual wellness and this is probably why my parents didn't know how strong my faith is until they read my CaringBridge page. I'm not sure why I've been so private about it, maybe it's because of society. Sometimes I have the feeling that people shy away from those who have a strong faith, like maybe it will be pushed on them (now this is just my opinion – right or wrong) and I was one that always worried about what people thought of me. Since I've been going through this journey of CANcer, I decided that I am just going to be me and not hide in the shadows. I need to quit worrying about what everyone else thinks and focus on what I believe in. Life is too short. I don't want to have any regrets in life. I am still the same person I was before, just more vocal in my values, views of life, and spirituality.

 Romans 8:28 ~ All things work together for good for those who love the Lord.

STILL GOING STRONG

Be confident. Too many days are wasted comparing ourselves to others and wishing to be something we aren't. Everybody has their own strengths and weaknesses, and it is only when you accept everything you are – and aren't – that you will truly succeed.

~ Unknown

As days went by in the confined space of those hospital walls, a nurse asked if I would be willing to speak to a young man who received the same diagnosis as I had. He was on his third day of chemo so I was a bit ahead of him in the process. I thought about how scared and nervous I had felt those first few days – and even as the time wore on – and desperately wanted to help him if I could. Before I went to his room, I copied down a prayer that I read often (more than once a day) to remind me of God's healing power and love. I strongly feel this prayer has been a huge help in healing me as I trudge through muddy waters in search of restoration. Just as a water lily comes up through the dark, murky, and dirty shallow waters in order to bloom into a magnificent beautiful flower, I've been envisioning myself as that same magnificent water lily. Slowly, one day at a time, one colored clip at a time, coming up through that dark water, until the completion of radiance and wholeness.

The prayer that helped me in this journey is taken from *God's Creative Power Gift Collection* by Charles Capps. "Christ has redeemed me from the curse of the law. Therefore, I forbid any sickness or disease to come upon this body. Every disease germ and every virus that touches this body dies instantly in the name of Jesus. Every organ and every tissue of this body functions in the perfection to which God created it to function, and I forbid any malfunction in this body, in the name of Jesus." (Gal. 3:13, Rom. 8:11, Gen. 1:31, Matt. 16:19.)

When I arrived at the patient's room, I told him that I wasn't trying to push anything on him, but if he would read this prayer anytime he was feeling down, nervous, scared, or when he didn't feel like he could muster the strength needed to endure the side effects of chemo, he might notice a positive shift or change beginning to occur. For me, the more I read this prayer, the more my heart believed in its message, the more open I became to miracles showing up in my life. I also gave him my CaringBridge website information in the event he wanted to read about my experiences with chemo. I showed him a photo of my family and told him that they were the reason I continued to fight for my life and he must find a reason to live as well.

It's so difficult to feel normal when you are in a situation like this – on chemo twenty-four hours a day, not knowing what will come next – so I tried to comfort him by distracting him a bit with some stories and we had some laughs. I didn't stay long because I know how tiring chemo treatments can be, but was so glad I met him. He was younger than me by a few years, with his whole life ahead of him. I wished him the very best and reminded him that I would be lifting him up in prayer, too.

After I left his room, I was making my usual rounds walking around the hospital. I began a habit of walking around the hospital when I was feeling strong enough for it. I ran into a beautiful woman (probably around the age of sixty) that I had briefly spoken to before. She and her husband were sitting in the breezeway, looking at Dodge Street in silence, as I passed them on my walk. I said hello and the woman asked how I was doing and what condition I had. I told her my diagnosis, but also shared that I believed the chemo had worked. I strongly thought and felt in my heart that I was in remission. I was just waiting for the data to prove it.

She told me that she began her journey with cervical cancer but found that it had spread. In fact, when she was in surgery to remove the tumors, the doctors saw that they had infiltrated too many areas of her body and immediately closed her up. She said they would be leaving the hospital in about five days to go home to start hospice. Boy, that was a tough conversation. Her husband said he was so worried to go home with her in the event he didn't know what to do to help her at any given time.

I desperately wanted to comfort the couple and reassure them in some small way. I reminded them that we all have untapped strength inside of us that reacts to tough situations when needed. I believe that God gives us the courage and wherewithal to get through even the scariest of times. He has been with me this entire time, wrapping me in love and strength.

 Psalm 107:19-20 ~ Then they cried to the Lord in their trouble, and he saved them in their distress. He sent his Word and healed them; He rescued them from the grave.

In Remission

It's August 29, and I was just informed by my doctor that the chemo treatment was effective and I am in full remission. Praise the Lord! The entire time my doctor was talking, my hands were folded in prayer close to my heart, with a huge smile on my face, just anticipating the results. I whole-heartedly felt that I was in remission because I can breathe easier and I don't have swollen lymph nodes, or night sweats anymore... like my health is restoring each and every day.

I will be allowed to go home when my blood counts are high enough, making sure I go in for lab work regularly in the event I need blood transfusions or platelets during this recovery period. At this point, I only have a few chemo treatments left and they will be four weeks apart from each other. I will be in the hospital for approximately a week during each phase of treatment. My doctor still wants my brother, Matt, to go to Nebraska Medicine to see if he is a perfect match in the event that I need a stem cell transplant. The stem cell transplant option is Plan B, but we need to be ready. I'm a little nervous about this option because there is a thirty percent chance of mortality and possibility of lifelong health issues if my body reacts to or rejects the transplant. Of course, at this moment we are not at a place to be considering Plan B, so for now I am focusing on Plan A. I'm thankful that Matt is coming in for the tests, so we are prepared for all options. I pray he is a match. The risk factor decreases if a sibling is able to give their stem cells.

 Romans 12:12 ~ Rejoice in hope, be patient in tribulation, be constant in prayer.

TOUGH RECOVERY

*May God grant you always...A sunbeam to warm you,
a moonbeam to charm you, a sheltering angel so nothing
can harm you. Laughter to cheer you. Faithful friends near you.
And whenever you pray, Heaven to hear you.*

~ Irish Blessing

It's August 31, and the past couple of days have been very tough. I find myself feeling emotional at times. It's one thing to beat CANcer, but another to move forward with the side effects of chemo. Some days I experience deep, deep sadness, and while in my mind I know that I need to keep a positive outlook, I also know that I cannot ignore the sadness and fear I am feeling. I thought this part would be easier. I didn't expect to experience so much physical pain. And this is really saying something for me because I feel like I have always been one to tolerate pain well.

Currently, a nurse gives me a daily shot in my torso to jump-start the production of white blood cells. Just thinking about this shot makes me a little anxious because the shot is painful and the medicine itself stings as it makes its way through my body. And this happens every day until my blood counts begin to rise. I use ice packs before I receive the shot in an effort to numb the area and that seems to help. It's not just the pain of the shot when I receive it, though. It seems that everything I undergo these days comes with additional side effects. One of the side effects of this particular shot is that my bones ache afterward because of the 'jumpstart' production of white blood cells. I really didn't have a conception of what it would feel like for my bones to ache before all of this. Now, I have no questions about that.

Yesterday, I needed two units of blood. When I have received blood in the past, I seemed to get energy shortly afterward, but this time, I had a different reaction, along with a fever. On top of all that, my body ached all over. It was very difficult to get comfortable and sleep. I have found that Tylenol reduces the pain significantly for a short while, but I can only have so much of it in one day, due to the possibility of it affecting my liver. I was also told that my potassium was low. This can cause body aches as well. I was so glad potassium supplements were prescribed and am hoping this will alleviate the pain.

My platelets are low as well, and my menstrual cycle is very heavy. This is scary because I soaked the bed through my pad in a short amount of time yesterday. I was given two units of platelets and had a fever off and on throughout the process. Fortunately, the bleeding is much lighter now and I am hoping it subsides soon. I don't want to risk bleeding out, as my platelets are so low right now. I've been told that there are about thirty thousand platelets in a unit. I can't believe how low my numbers get. They absorb into my body quickly.

I have been taking a pill to prevent me from having a menstrual cycle since I've been admitted because I don't have the clotting power to stop bleeding if it gets out of hand, so far it hasn't worked. My gynecologist stopped by again today to visit with me about other options. I am now taking an estrogen pill for the next few days and praying this helps.

A Few Days Later

My blood pressure continues to rise. I had been averaging 130/60, but then it jumped to 143/93 and my concern grew. I thought I was having another allergic reaction to a medication, and was relieved when the infectious disease doctor came last night. He is remarkable and assured me that I was not reacting to the new medication given, but he did check all my oral medications and found out what was causing hypertension (high blood pressure). The pill I had been taking to stop my menstrual cycle caused hypertension so my doctor prescribed another medication to lower my blood pressure. This morning, I am at 126/77. I told the medical care team that I was not going to take medication to suppress my menstrual cycle anymore. No one tells you about how all of these medications might interact and cause other side effects. And there are so many side effects! Chemo side effects, medications to help with the chemo side effects and then medications to help with the side effects from those medications. It makes my head spin at times and brings up these emotions that I didn't realize I was even harboring.

For the past few days, I've had severe sciatica nerve pain that shoots down my left leg. I don't know if it was from the bone marrow biopsy itself, or if it was due to the way I was positioned during the biopsy. It was an awkward position for me to lay and my muscles did tense up during the procedure when I could feel the stinging of the shots and pressure while they were gathering bone marrow and taking a bone fragment. One of my health care providers demonstrated some easy exercises that I can do to naturally help my back return to the proper placement – if, in fact, that is the reason for my pain – but I am not sure it's working very well yet. I am also supposed to alternate ice packs and heat pads on my buttocks and leg. Please pray that God works His magic and gives me relief from this terrible pain. If the pain localizes in the biopsy area then I need to have an MRI to check for a hematoma (buildup of blood).

I have also been suffering from a terrible rash on my trunk area, back, arms, and legs. At least the rash doesn't itch or bother me. I was prescribed a cream to put on the area three times a day. They think it's due to the Hibiclens skin cleanser to keep germs to a minimum. I've had to use it in the shower since I got here on August 13. I was told to stop using the

Hibiclens and get a moisturizing liquid soap. Tim bought me a gentle liquid soap, but this is day two with the new soap and I still have a terrible rash.

As if all of that isn't enough, I have this sharp pain and hot spot on my arm where my PICC line is located. The doctor ordered a Doppler test to see if I had a blood clot. Luckily, they did not find one. It is assumed that my tetanus shot (given just days before my diagnosis) is still giving me trouble, so I continue to put ice on the area.

I have also continued to suffer from pain in my stomach area and was told that my liver enzymes were elevated. My doctor thought it was in my best interest to check for an enlarged liver, as well as other organ damage by means of an ultrasound. Fortunately, the results of the ultrasound and all my organs are functioning as they should be. Interestingly enough, they found that I have an extra spleen (called an accessory spleen) during the ultrasound. Accessory spleens are found in about ten percent of the population and are small in size. Typically, they do not cause harm. One of the personnel said that spleens contain white blood cells and fight infecting germs in the blood. They also control the level of blood cells and remove damaged red blood cells. Good thing I have two spleens then! I don't consider this as an imperfection of my body, but instead, I see it as a lifesaver. Spleens play an important role in protecting our bodies from illness.

With all of these difficulties this week I have been letting the emotions flow as much as I can while also trying to keep a positive outlook. It's difficult when you are feeling both physical pain and fear at the same time. I find when we are feeling good we take that for granted. For the majority of my life, I have been healthy and strong. It never occurred to me that my body would go through something like this when I was feeling good. These days, though, it's tough to remember what it even feels like to not have pain and fear running through my body.

This week, even with all of these struggles and challenges, I am leaning on God and my faith as much as I possibly can. I know that I cannot do this alone. I've had my prayer shawl wrapped around me tightly and continue to plead for a full recovery. One of the health care providers came to see me this evening. I told him that I was still having some issues with my sciatic nerve today, but that I had fallen asleep with my prayer shawl wrapped around me and when I woke up, all of the pain was gone. When my doctor was getting ready to leave, he said, "Use prayer shawl as needed, doctor's orders." I chuckled and said, "You got it!"

The Christian songs that continuously play in my hospital room have really helped me. Even as a young child, music had a way of comforting me; not only because of its upbeat rhythm but also from the lyrics that were significantly impactful or relatable to my personal life. When I was nine or ten years old, I remember choreographing my own dance moves to the albums of Madonna, Huey Lewis and the News, and Mister Mister songs, while energetically singing along in my backyard or driveway. Oftentimes, I would make my family watch me proudly perform an act.

As I grew up, music continued to have an effect on me and helped me through difficult personal situations. Music got me through break-ups and while I wept from the loss of young love. Songs were there for happy times, too. In fact, my friends and I would sing melodies while walking around the town, just for fun. Music also presented a way for me to release deep-rooted feelings that I wasn't prepared to share with anyone else. I would write it on paper and tuck it away in the depths of my dark closet until the next time I felt the need to privately express myself. I'm sure many can relate. It presents an immediate way of stirring up emotions that need to be released or received.

I feel so blessed for all that God has done and continues to do for me. I'm overwhelmed with grace and gratitude to see Him at work, by allowing miracles to happen for my highest good and letting me know that He is with me every step of the way. Prayers mean the world to me and have helped me get through this phase of recovery without a doubt. God hears all the prayers and cries for help. I know He has a plan for me and I hold that beautiful plan – whatever it is – in my heart and mind as I look forward to the months of recovery in front of me.

 Joshua 1:9 ~ Have I not commanded you? Be strong and courageous. Do not be afraid; do not be discouraged, for the Lord your God will be with you wherever you go.

TRUST THE SIGNS

God whispers to us in our pleasures,
speaks in our consciences, but shouts in our pains.
It is His megaphone to rouse a deaf world.

~ C.S. Lewis

For the past several days, maybe even a week, I have been praying for a rainbow. To me, rainbows are a sign that God is with me. I believe it's His way of saying, "Mary, I'm embracing you with my love. I will take care of you." Rainbows bring me great joy – even when it's just a fraction that shines through dispersed clouds in the sky. That being the case, it had been storming most of those days, and I'm not talking about a little bit of rain, I'm talking about a downpour – and the storm outside reminds me of the storm inside my body that I am navigating. So often, after the storm, the sun comes out, the world feels fresh and a rainbow appears, promising hope. This is what I had been praying for.

Nearly a week after my request and a couple days ago, my aunt texted me. She congratulated me on the great news of remission I have received and she told me that she had felt that I was in remission before we officially heard. She sent another text with several hearts all with different colors. In the text, she wrote, "Here's your rainbow. I'm excited for you!" My aunt lives in a different state and travels a lot for work. She had no idea that it had been raining here or that I even wanted to see a rainbow. In fact, no one did – it's not something I talk about very much because it feels like a sacred message between me and God. However, this time I couldn't resist. I wrote back, "Funny, I have been praying to see a rainbow for the past few days. You just gave me what I've been wanting through a text!" My aunt said, "That was the Holy Spirit and just another sign of God's great love. He can send a rainbow in the most unexpected ways." Ahh, yes – the lesson of expectation. I was EXPECTING my rainbow to come a certain way, but in the end, I still received it. And because it was through someone whom I dearly love and came with hearts, it meant even more.

I love my rainbow of hearts. Hearts are also special to me. I collect heart-shaped rocks. Why? I enjoy walking outdoors. Over the years, I have gone on many walks and talked to God about everything under the sun – the good, bad, and everything in between. Sometimes we converse together in my mind and other times, I speak out loud – with passion, tears, laughs, and triumph. In my heart, I've always known that God is with me, but I desired a tangible experience between us – A way for me to know that He is with me. I wanted to think of a way for this to happen that was out of the ordinary, or at least not something that a person would 'see' every day. I began to ask God to give me a sign by placing heart-shaped rocks in my path as a way for us to communicate, especially during those times that hearing him may be obscured with environmental and mental noise. I began to notice heart-shaped rocks on my graveled lane while walking. I would pick up each 'rock of love' and put it in my pocket, later storing it in a clear jar – my jar of hearts, placed where I can see it. Sometimes, I even recognize heart shapes in other objects, such as clouds. Whenever I find a heart-shaped rock, cloud, or another object, I feel like it's a message from God, reminding me that He is with me always. So, to receive a rainbow of hearts is indeed something very special and something I will save for myself. I really needed that.

 Isaiah 41:10 ~ So do not fear, for I am with you; do not be dismayed, for I am your God. I will strengthen you and help you; I will uphold you with my righteous right hand.

AN EYE-OPENING

A house is made with walls and beams;
a home is built with love and dreams.

~ Ralph Waldo Emerson

It seemed like a dream, only I knew it was reality. I was given permission to go home because my white blood count was high enough. I can still feel the rush of emotions coming in like a strong tidal wave from the ocean while reflecting on my last few hours in the hospital on September 4. I can't adequately describe the overwhelming feeling of gratitude I have right now. Just thinking about breathing fresh outdoor air sends a rush of adrenaline throughout my body, as if the car ride home won't be thrilling enough. I know it will be the best ride ever! You know the kind – when you see a beautiful dog with his head out the window, mouth open wide, and his ears flying in the wind – that kind!

When I first came to the hospital, I didn't know if or when I would be coming home. I keep thinking about what I want to do first when at home and the answer is simple: Cuddle with all my children and Tim on the couch, feel the love, and just breathe. Oh, and I can't forget about our dog, Rick! I miss him, too. Animals don't always receive the credit they deserve. They love us so unconditionally and provide such a sense of calm and acceptance. At the moment, I don't have a lot of energy and feel very tired most of the time, but I am determined to go for short walks, as I can tolerate them.

If I have learned anything from this journey, it is that I need to listen to what my body is telling me... overexertion and recovery, as much as I hate to admit it, don't seem to be an optimal combination. In an attempt to satisfy this restraint, my current goal is to make mindful movements – accepting my limitations in whatever forms they present themselves, but not underestimating my abilities from the get-go. Every day is different, meaning the demands of my body will never remain constant, but it's comforting to know that my strength will grow with time. I will not have to worry about pushing myself too hard for much longer. I am committed to honoring this. When I first came to the hospital, I didn't know if or when I would be coming home. It was a frightening time. Now, I am almost to the point of breaking out of this joint! Don't get me wrong, I have had the greatest care from the medical care team to make my stay the best it could possibly be, but that line from Dorothy in *The Wizard of Oz*, "There's no place like home," is a cliche for a reason – it's true! I feel like my recovery will multiply when I'm at home.

Ahh, I can hear it clearly, the sound of freedom is chiming loudly in my ears. I believe I've taken my independence for granted because, frankly, it has never been taken away until a few weeks ago. Even though my wish of returning home came true – and is happening on the special day that Tim and I married fifteen years ago – the thought of leaving the hospital is scary, too. I am in a sterile environment here and it keeps the risks of me catching an illness to a minimum. Of course, I am fearful about getting sick from my children, but I also desperately want to be at home with them. An internal conflict to say the least! I do know, though, that God will watch over us during this time and take care of all our needs. And my doctor reminded me that my blood counts are better now than they were before I came to the hospital. Hearing that sent me back to a place of sincere gratitude for all the blessings that came with this frightening diagnosis. I was *really* sick and found myself grasping onto any shred of hope to make it through. My blood counts are not where they should be yet, but I know they will get there!

Shortly after my doctor left, another nurse came with bags so I could begin packing all the things that contributed to keeping my spirits up while there. The idea of gathering items to take home was nostalgic. I remember hanging my family picture on the wall, across from where I laid in bed for many weeks, so I could easily remind myself why I was in this fight for my life. I also had a picture of my parents and my grandmother in the same vicinity to remind me of my strength and that all things are possible through Christ, which is what I was raised to believe. There was a beautiful drawing of a woman who was bald (representing me), hanging next to my family photo. It had been sketched by my thirteen-year-old niece to remind me that I AM A SURVIVOR, as the shirt stated. And how could I forget to mention the "G.I. Mary Jane" banner that I read on a daily basis? The photo evoked courageous images in my mind and helped me persevere on those tough days – when I just wanted to stop the clock of time and have some relief of pain. There was a multitude of cards, letters, and well wishes to gather too. All of these items meant a great deal to me and I will forever treasure them.

When the nurse was getting ready to leave my room, she asked if I would like to go for one last walk in the hall with her. I said, "Sure, let me grab my mask." From day one at the hospital, I was not to leave my room without covering my face with a mask to protect me from germs. She told me that I didn't need my mask anymore, that I was going home and could walk the halls without it. This news was difficult for me to wrap my head around. The fact that I had to wear a mask outside my room yesterday, but I didn't today was bizarre. What if I got sick from taking a final winner's lap without a mask? My eyes started to fill up with emotional tears on our walk. It had been so long since I had been free from covering my face with a mask. My nurse chuckled and said there were extra Kleenexes in her office that we could grab as we made the round. However, I composed myself and proudly walked around my usual stretch in the hallway. Nurses were clapping, congratulating me, and sending well wishes for my much-deserved time at home. I saw some of the patients (who became my friends) that were admitted after me – still hooked up to their IV carts. We exchanged phone numbers so we could stay in touch and be of support for each other.

When Tim arrived at the hospital, we were just waiting for one more doctor to give me the approval to go home. Tim ran a few loads to the car so we would be able to leave upon discharge. I decided to go to my special friend's room to say goodbye one last time (for now). She came to the hospital two days prior to my arrival and was also leaving the same day as me. We are both in remission! I remember being so scared for what was to come and then I met her, a stranger in the hall. We quickly became familiars, oftentimes having lengthy conversations on our hallway walks. She gave me a sense of peace. You see, this woman (age of 59) had beaten cancer three previous times (thyroid twice, breast once) and now was fighting a fourth, acute myeloid leukemia. She was such a true inspiration to me. Her attitude was remarkable and she gave me tips, such as, 'Make sure you clean your room daily with sanitizing wipes and wash your hands often to lower risks of infection and sickness. A lot of patients get sick and this helps alleviate other complications.' I wouldn't have thought to wipe my room down, but I listened to what this wise woman had to say and had a strong feeling that she played a role in my overall health while here. God brings people in and out of our life so we can help each other evolve, even when we don't realize it at the moment. During our time at the hospital, we helped each other through the tough times when we were able to leave our rooms and meet up in the hallway, but there were times both of us were not feeling well enough to visit. I hope she will be back at the hospital around the same time I return too. Regardless, both of us are going through this fight and we have every intention of beating this for lifelong remission.

We reached the main doors to exit the hospital and I was overwhelmed with emotions when the sun hit my skin and the outside breeze brushed against my face. I took a deep breath in, and looked up to the sky with a smile. It was beyond words to feel and see all of God's creations in a new light. It was as if all of my senses were fully expanded and I was actually 'seeing' the world in all of its glory for the first time. It became clear to me that my field of vision had magnified sometime during my stay in the hospital. The entire trip home, I was just soaking in all the freedom, while penetrating the deeper understanding of my new perspective within my soul. I thanked God for allowing me another day, and hopefully many more years. I couldn't wait to get home and just be.

Secure At Home

Driving down the long lane to reach my home was humbling. The trees were swaying gracefully in sync with the light breeze. Squirrels were playfully scurrying along the grassy area and around the trees. There was a bunny (I often see several during long walks on our acreage) sitting in the tall grass, as still as a statue when we pulled into the lane. Warm thoughts of my maternal grandmother came to mind, as she always does when I see bunnies on my walks at home. Funny as it may sound, I believe this is a way for my grandma to let me know that she is still with me, even in the afterlife. Generally, the bunnies sit calmly, gazing in my direction, as if we have a connection and this feeling of unconditional love sweeps over me. I respond lightheartedly – sometimes even speaking briefly to my grandma – and continue on the path, with anticipation for another encounter. I'd like to think that anything is possible in the afterlife. This fun game that I call, 'going on a bunny hunt,' has actually become the highlight of my walking experiences. I look forward to spotting them and didn't realize just how much this incidental occurrence meant to me until now.

We pulled into the driveway and I couldn't wait to step into my home. The house that I had left almost a month prior was in front of me. When I walked into our house, familiar sights and smells surrounded me. The house was so clean and it felt absolutely incredible to be back. The kids were still at school for another three hours, so it was very quiet and felt a little empty. There was a load of laundry on the couch that needed to be folded. I never thought there would be a day that I actually wanted to fold clothes, but this delighted me so much! I made neat piles of all the kids' freshly folded clothes so they could put them away when they got home.

Tim and I went to my parents' house later in the afternoon to meet the kids there. My mom picked them up from the bus stop, as usual. My kids didn't know that I was home because I wasn't certain on the exact day and didn't want to disappoint them. When I saw them, it was unquestionably the highlight of my month to see their faces light up and be able to hug them all! Of course, it was bittersweet to see my parents and brother too. It was an emotional time. We ate dinner at my parents' house, took some photos, and stayed for a movie. The evening was perfect!

When we arrived home and got the kids settled into bed, I took a moment to thank God for all that He has done to return me safely to my family. Every now and then, I shed a few joyful tears for all the works that God performed for me. I have a strong feeling that my time on earth is not over yet and He will get me through all the chemo treatments and allow me to remain in remission for long life... I have to rely on FAITH!

Lunchtime Epiphany

September 9, was the first day that I had to go to the Methodist Estabrook Cancer Center to get my blood levels checked since being discharged from the hospital just a few days prior. After my blood was drawn, I was to remain in the waiting room at my doctor's office for results. Fortunately, all my blood work looked well enough for me to leave without a transfusion this time. It was a good feeling to leave the office on a high note.

My aunt (my driver) and I went out to eat lunch afterward and had a lot of laughs. Funny, I wore a scarf over my head the entire day and felt more comfortable than I would have with a hot, itchy wig on. I didn't feel like people were staring at me or that they felt sorry for me. I was free to be me! After some thought, I wondered how people could feel sorry for someone who is full of life and having a great time laughing and reminiscing with another loved one anyway? During our lunch date, I realized that I don't need a wig to maintain a normal-looking persona. There was no awkwardness that came from our time out in public. In fact, I didn't feel any different than the group sitting next to us. I was okay with the way I looked and did not feel the need to hide behind fake hair.

Redefining Value

Now that I've been home for over a week, it has been remarkable to spend more time with my family. It's becoming clear that our life was centered around crazy schedules and deadlines before. Everything was so rushed and programmed. I didn't have time to recognize that I was missing out on special moments and simplicity because it was difficult enough just to stay afloat. Capturing the real meaning of living with purpose was not in sight. Maybe the only way I could discover this epiphany was to have gone through the cancer experience. It forced me to slow down and reassess what mattered most.

I love all the little things that I may have taken for granted before... like my youngest, Shaylee, singing a made-up song so innocently while she is playing (when she doesn't think anyone is listening). She is such a happy child and always has been. When I'm at home, I usually don't have my head covered because it is more comfortable (unless I get cold). Oftentimes, Shaylee will come up to me, stare at my bald head and say, "Mom, you are beautiful and your eyes are so pretty!" It just melts my heart because I know she is so curious about my hair, but refrains from talking about it constantly. When I was in the hospital and we FaceTimed, Shaylee would always ask about my hair and what color I think it will be when it grows back.

She is so comical! In the evenings, she sits on my lap and gives my arms kisses, telling me how much she loves me.

Brody, my oldest, is so kind-hearted and asks for quick hugs throughout the day to show he cares, then goes about his business as usual. Holly, my second oldest is such a tremendous help! She is a mini-me and always willing to lend a hand with the younger two so I can rest peacefully. Then there's Colby. He tells me that I'm the best mom in the world and he loves me so much, while wrapping his arms firmly around me. As I reflect on the past several weeks, I have a better understanding of what freedom means to me. I aim to consciously spend quality time with my family and genuinely experience every part of their intricate being. I don't want to get sucked back into a self-absorbed, unfulfilled life, surrounded by materialistic items, and missing out on what's most important. And I will do my best to preserve this new vantage point.

 Galatians 5:1 ~ It is for freedom that Christ has set us free. Stand firm, then, and do not let yourselves be burdened again by a yoke of slavery.

HOME AWAY FROM HOME

You can have more than one home. You can carry
your roots with you, and decide where they grow.

~ Henning Mankell

Driving to the hospital for blood work on September 11, made me a little anxious. I was prepared for my calcium levels to be elevated and I knew that I would need fluids if they hadn't decreased. However, I was more nervous about what I didn't know about my blood results than what I was prepared for. Upon arriving at Methodist Estabrook Cancer Center, I had my blood drawn and then while Tim and I waited for my results, we went to visit my young friend who was in the Methodist Hospital next door.

It was great to see my friend! He is done with chemo and has already had his bone marrow biopsy. He is anxiously waiting for the results to find out if he is in remission. I know that feeling all too well. In fact, it seems like CANcer is often a series of waiting games, but the games are not fun. At every turn, each wait for results feels like it is longer than the last, and there is nothing you can do to speed up the process. I pray that he has received the news by now and that the results were in his favor. I've been on the receiving end of those good results too and nothing feels better!

I also loved seeing all the nurses that were caring for me while I was in the hospital just a few short days ago. They were so nice and couldn't believe how good I looked since leaving a week ago – no more rashes all over my body (except my legs), the color in my face has returned, and I have put on a few pounds (yes, already!). There's something to say about being home.

When we were done visiting with everyone, I returned to the doctor's office to get my results. I was hoping for the best but was disappointed when the nurse told me that my white blood cells were dropping faster than they would like to see. When I left the hospital a week ago, my white counts were very high because of the shots I received, so I wasn't as nervous to be in a few public situations for short periods. I need to be more cautious now. At least my calcium levels were in the normal range.

The nurse made an appointment for me to go to the hospital on Sunday morning for more blood work in the event that I need a transfusion or another shot in my stomach to bring my white blood count up. They did not want to wait until Monday since my levels were dropping fast. For now, all I can do is pray for my highest good, and that's enough.

 James 1:2-4 ~ Count it all joy, my brothers, when you meet trials of various kinds, for you know that the testing of your faith produces steadfastness. And let steadfastness have its full effect, that you may be perfect and complete, lacking in nothing.

DO NOT COMPARE

She was powerful not because she wasn't scared but because she went on so strongly, despite the fear.

~ Atticus

 Psalm 30:2 states: "O Lord my God, I called to you for help and you healed me."

I am STRONG, and I am a SURVIVOR.

As I continue on this road, I am trying my best not to let fear take over my life, but sometimes I become a little paranoid. When one of my children sneezes, coughs, or has a stuffy nose, fear rears its ugly head. Sometimes even though they are trying so hard, my children aren't as cautious as I would like. They don't always cover their mouths and wash their hands, and I need to explain to them that yes, I beat CANcer, but my immune system is weak, and I will not let an illness defeat me. I realize this is difficult for kids to understand. Everything is so immediate when you are young. And their mom is here now, so they don't always equate their actions as being contributors to my health and well-being. It's complicated for sure!

On Sunday, September 14, my brother Matt took me to the hospital. After the blood was drawn and we were waiting to hear back from the doctor, Matt and I went to visit my young friend – with the same diagnosis as me – who was still in the hospital. It's nice to have those connections with other patients and visit about some commonalities. Although, I have been told that you cannot equate yourself to anyone with the same condition because not all bodies are alike and may not respond to chemo the same. There are just so many variables when dealing with any kind of CANcer for any one person, that it's like comparing apples to oranges. Also, some people go into the hospital sicker than others. That's understandable.

I was hoping to hear that my friend was in remission just like me, but was disappointed to see that he had a chemo bag hanging from his IV cart when we walked into his room. I didn't say anything about it until he brought it up. I knew that he had another seven days of chemo, just like the first round we both received. We talked about lots of different things and how we are going to get through this. He is almost there and will be ready for the shots to bring his white blood counts up at the end of next week. I can't wait to hear about his reaction when he finally gets out of the hospital and rediscovers the freedom he had before entering. I continue to pray for him and my other friends going through this.

When the doctor called me, I was so grateful to God that I did not need a blood transfusion once again. My red blood cells had dropped since Thursday, but were not low enough for me to get a transfusion.

The ride home was great! Matt and I jammed out to rock music from the '80s because he said we needed to celebrate (while giving me a high five). It's funny, I hadn't heard the CD he played in years, but still remembered all the words. Driving in the car with Matt, and the music loud brought back so many memories. On rare occasions, Matt would let me go cruising with him on the main drag in our hometown, sometimes with his friends, and other times it was just the two of us. Matt would loudly play all the cool songs with the top off his scout or blazer (whatever car he owned at the time). We would sing along, as the wind blew through my long sandy blonde hair. I'd have a huge smile on my face. I felt special. It seemed as though time slowed down briefly and there was not a care in the world. I love spending time with Matt and don't get the chance to often because of the long distance between us.

I go back to the clinic on Tuesday for more lab work, then have an appointment with my doctor. I will most likely find out when they want me to return to the hospital for my next round of chemo and when they want my brother to get tested to see if he is a match for a stem cell transplant.

I am praying I won't have to go that route in the end. I was told if a transplant was needed and works as it should, it would be the best option for me. However, if my body rejects it, there is the possibility of health issues for a lifetime, that is IF a person survives. I will continue to pray for the best scenario. That's all I can do.

I decided to go for a walk when Matt dropped me off at home. It was very peaceful outside. The dogs were following me around while sniffing the ground. It was nice to take some time to thank God for all His works in my life, the blessings that He has given me, and just gaze at all the beauty surrounding me. It feels so good to be alive!

 Psalms 28:7 ~ The LORD is my strength and my shield; My heart trusts in Him, and I am helped; Therefore my heart exults, and with my song, I shall thank Him.

TWO

FAITH IS RISING

Holding onto faith and hope while praying for new beginnings is challenging. When the reality of my CANcer set in, I told myself that I must fight for every breath and believe in all possibilities. I asked God to let me know where to go from there. He continues to show me the way, and I now understand the importance of searching for the peace within your struggle.

BLISTERS ON MY FEET

The ocean is everything I want to be.
Beautiful, mysterious, wild, and free.

~ Unknown

I had an appointment with my doctor on September 16. He asked how things were going at home and how my mood was in general. Things are going well, but I get tired quickly, especially in the late afternoon. I need to remember to take it easy.

Tim and I are doing our best to keep our kids' lives as normal as possible, despite the current struggles with each week-long round of chemo. If all goes according to plan, my last round will be in early January 2015. After that, the possibilities are endless! Each day we are given is a gift from God, and I intend to make the most of it.

I've had blisters on my feet since the beginning of the school year on August 7, and I'm finally starting to notice that they are healing. Back then, I wanted to look nice, so I had complimented each of my outfits with the perfect pair of heels. Tennis shoes or flats just wouldn't do! In my defense, I also didn't know how sick I was until August 12. Had I known that I was so ill, I would have made better decisions to care for my feet.

It took me back nine years ago to a time when my friend and I were both pregnant, each with our third child. It was a scorching day in July, and I only had a few more weeks before my baby boy was to arrive. My friend was due in October, so she was not as far along in her pregnancy. Our families were at the annual John C. Fremont Days festival that spans several blocks in the town. Everyone enjoys all the sights, merchandise, and events held during the three-day celebration.

I wanted to be comfortable that day, so I wore a maternity shirt, shorts, and tennis shoes. I knew it would be a long day walking in the hot summer heat. My friend wore this beautiful dress and high heels! As the day continued, I was getting tired – along with my feet – so I asked my friend, "How are you doing? Do your feet hurt?" I will never forget what she said to me, "Yes, they are killing me, but remember, fashion before comfort!" To this day, I think of that reply and laugh about it. At the beginning of

August, I was one of the many that chose fashion before comfort! I'm sure there are a few who can relate. But from where I sit now, the comfort looks far more appealing and makes a lot more sense.

Now that my platelets are closer to the normal range and still rising, my blisters are finally healing from the high heels I wore in early August. All I can do is laugh because I was even prescribed a cream for them in the hospital. My orders were to apply it two to three times a day to prevent infection, as the blisters on my feet refused to heal because my platelets were so low.

Let's face it: Women want to feel beautiful. When I walk out of my house, I want my look to represent how I feel on the inside. Nice clothing boosts my confidence, aligns my posture, and increases my disposition. If I have the appearance of strength, I am ready to conquer the world! This frame of mind positively affects my overall attitude and demeanor. It builds my self-esteem and refines my life.

Having said all of this, I often wonder why women feel like they need to live up to the veneer of perfection. When did this all begin? And what was the cause? Is the media to blame? Perhaps some of it, well, maybe the majority of it. Models and movie stars need to have a specific look to make it in the field. Even magazines display the perfect woman: The right size, height, and facial characteristics. But how much of this is real, and what cost do these models pay? Some women go to extreme measures to meet society's expectations by undergoing cosmetic surgery or limiting their food intake. Technology advances have made it easy to conceal blemishes or accentuate features. Children see this on a daily basis, which has a significant impact on their perception of themselves and others.

I see something growing in our world, although it has been around for a while. With all this emphasis on perfection, I notice how often girls (in particular) feel the need to compete with each other and make harsh comparisons. Why do some feel the need to beat others down? Does that *really* make them feel better about themselves?

I believe those who hurt others are also wounded inside and possibly have a hefty load of demands placed on their shoulders. Maybe they have been verbally attacked themselves, and that's the only way they know how to behave. We don't live in the shoes of others and have not traveled on the same road. The mirror of social media gives us the means to portray a reflection of flawlessness instead of representing life as it truly is. Every post we create provides us with an opportunity to curate which images we want the world to see. This fantasy representation may give the impression of inferiority. Don't let yourself get stuck in a rabbit hole of fabricated stories. In the world we live in, perfection doesn't exist.

 Psalm 139:14 ~ I praise you because I am fearfully and wonderfully made; your works are wonderful, I know that full well.

JUST A SWINGIN'

The world's a playground. You know that when you are a kid,
but somewhere along the way everyone forgets it.

~ Zooey Deschanel as Allison (*Yes Man*, 2008)

There's something about swaying back and forth on a swing that makes me smile. It may be due to the breeze that gently sweeps against my skin as I move back and forth through the air. Perhaps it's also the excitement of gliding rapidly through the open space and ascending toward the sky. I remember times when I felt especially brave and leaped off the swing to capture a brief rush, soaring through the air and landing gracefully (or not so gracefully) on the ground. Maybe it makes me smile for just one simple reason: It's fun! The swing allows me to remember how I felt as a child, gliding through the air without a care in the world.

I had an opportunity to witness my youngest daughter swinging at our house a few days ago during one of my walks. She looked so precious and was beaming from ear to ear! As I rounded the corner, Shaylee noticed I was watching her. She slowed down, tilted her head to the side, leaning it on one of the chains that held the swing, and was smiling at me. Her big brown eyes told me, "Come here, mom, and try this. It's fun!" So, after a few more laps, that's precisely what I did! I sat on a swing and began pumping my legs back and forth. Holly came over and asked what I was doing, most likely because it had been so long since I was even on a swing.

I told her that Shaylee looked like she was having fun, so I wanted to join her. Holly nodded with a crooked smile in agreement.

As I was pumping my legs back and forth, I really started focusing on the swinging and began to think about how much practice and perseverance it takes for a child to learn the mechanics of swinging independently. For most, it doesn't just come naturally. They must have the drive to gain proficiency; attitude plays an important role in mastering the skill. This concept can also apply to the skills of everyday life. If you find the reward favorable, you will be more determined to put forth the extra effort. Swinging is fun, so most kids want to learn how to do it.

Reflecting on my childhood experiences of these joyful moments of being carefree, I have to acknowledge that I did not miss out on any opportunities that came my way. When I moved to Chadron, Nebraska, in the middle of fifth grade, I left behind close friends. One friend, in particular, was what I would call 'my person' at the time. She and I had so many adventures together. She grew up in the country, so we had ample room to explore outdoors at her house. It wasn't uncommon for us to run through cornfields to arrive at our destination faster. We enjoyed paddle boating in the pond, chasing wild kittens in hopes of capturing one, swinging on her swing set, and including her dog (a border collie) on all of our adventures. We searched for canning jars for the insects we caught and poked holes in the lids to give them some air. On many occasions, the jar contained caterpillars, butterflies, fireflies, and even praying mantises as we examined them through the clear glass. After we finished inspecting our subjects, we set them free.

I was very sad when I had to move, but her family invited me to travel to California with them when I was in sixth grade. All I needed was spending money. It was a once-in-a-lifetime opportunity that I will forever be thankful for and will never forget. A few of our memorable activities included going to Knotts Berry Farm theme park, Disneyland, and Alcatraz Island. I had two hundred dollars of spending money, and the rest of the vacation was on their dime. That trip was one of the greatest highlights of my life. I used my money to buy gifts for each family member and purchased a couple of items for myself with the leftover cash. As the years passed, our friendship slowly fizzled. We don't keep in touch very often, but this friend will always be dear to my heart.

As I made friends in Chadron, it occurred to me that there *was* happiness beyond my parochial school. In the winter, my new friends and I would go sledding at Chadron State Park and warm up with a cup of hot cocoa and marshmallows afterward. We loved telling tales of our close calls with trees, brush, and boulders during our sledding escapade.

As the years progressed, I experienced even more firsts with these new companions. For instance, one of them invited me to go on an out-of-town skiing trip with her church's Youth Group. Additionally, in the spring, summer, and fall months, our friend group would always be out in nature: rock climbing, hiking on scenic trails, exploring forested areas, you name it! Another favorite activity was riding motorcycles and bicycles.

It was country living and slow-moving in my new town, and I was actually content. My dad and I even enjoyed fishing and shooting at targets when time allowed. Exposure to all these natural moments made a positive impact on my development. When there were times of trouble brewing in my life, and I wasn't able to find a solution with the help of friends, I leaned on nature to get me through.

Everything in life contributes to who you will become and what you are meant to be. Although a person's path consists of seemingly infinite encounters, life is short when it comes down to it. Sometimes, to make up for the fact that time seems to be moving so quickly, we try to cram as many activities into our days as possible. The flaw in this mindset is that we become distracted. When we pack our days with 'to-dos,' it's too easy to walk past and ignore opportunities. Don't lose sight of your passions in search of something better. Instead, keep an open mind when signs make themselves visible! I've begun to discover that slowing down just a bit and doing what I enjoy is the best way to mark my *own* path. And in doing so, the opportunities tend to find their way to me.

Chances will come as long as you remain aware. So, take a walk on the wild side and bring out your inner child! Try to remember what motivated you to learn from the very beginning. Joanne Raptis says it so purposefully, "Be like a tree. Stay grounded. Connect with your roots. Turn over a new leaf. Bend before you break. Enjoy your unique natural beauty. Keep growing."

Psalm 16:11 ~ You make known to me the path of life; you will fill me with joy in your presence, with eternal pleasures at your right hand.

LEAVES FALLING, FAITH RISING

Anyone who thinks fallen leaves are dead
has never watched them dancing on a windy day.

~ Shira Tamir

I often see yellow butterflies fluttering so gracefully around me on my walks outdoors. It's as if they are trying to relay the message that everything is going to be all right. God continues to give me signs of hope and reassures me that He is with me every step of the way. It feels *so* good to be alive, and I am grateful for every forward-moving step.

It's September 29, and on my walk today, I observed some leaves twirling delicately to the ground. As I watched these leaves falling, I began thinking about how specific events in our lives can cause us to fall. I don't mean to literally topple over, but to have an emotional fall. My most recent fall in life was when my doctor gave me this horrific diagnosis. I remember leaving the doctor's office with Tim, knowing that I had to tell my parents, brother, and children. It was devastating news for my family, but I reassured them that I would give the fight of my life to beat this dreadful disease because I had so much to live for.

We have all had trials in our lives at one time or another. It may be due to a falling out with a close friend, from a job that seems to be going nowhere, or possibly from the death of a loved one. Whatever the reason, it has a lasting effect. Generally, I want a 'quick fix' when I'm going through challenging times. So, I confide in my friends in hopes of good advice to help me find a solution to resolve the situation. Just having someone who will sit and listen to my problems almost always does the trick.

Friends have the advantage of an outsider's perspective when examining our issue. The holes in our dilemmas are much more clear from that vantage point. As humans, we are wired to simultaneously care for others and seek care for ourselves. This exchange is what keeps us going as a species. Our incredible capacity for compassion plays a pivotal role in our emotional wellness. With this being said, sometimes I forget to take my problems to God as well. I need to remember that He holds all the answers and presents all the solutions. I am learning this more and more as I grow in Christ.

Looking back on my current situation, perhaps I could have turned to God more than I did. But I take no shame in my actions. I did the best I could with the scenario I was given and welcomed my friends to stand beside me in this battle of the unknown. They were and continue to be a support system of positive encouragement. Occasionally, my patience is tested. But I'm content with the realization that God has perfect timing for all of us. We just need to pay close attention to the signs. Sometimes they hit you smack in the face, while other times, they are more subtle. Nevertheless, the signs are always there. You just need to look for them. If you aren't watchful, God's messages will fly right by.

Years ago, I was driving to work in the midst of one of my 'falls.' I noticed a van with a sticker on the back bumper. It said, "Got Faith?" I couldn't believe it. There it was, right in front of me! God gave me a sign to have faith and not worry over things I can't control (which I tend to do).

Additionally, a while back, I heard a story from one of Joyce Meyer Ministries radio podcasts, *Enjoying Everyday Life*. Joyce spoke of a donkey that falls into a pit. The story goes something like this: The donkey's owner, a farmer, heard his donkey crying in the pit, and he debated on whether or not to get him out because it would be a lot of work. The hole was deep, and the donkey was old. The farmer decided to gather some friends to help him bury the donkey. The men got shovels to fill the pit with dirt. As they were dumping shovelfuls of dirt on the donkey, it was making awful noises and bucking. It finally occurred to the donkey that if he just shook the dirt off his back, he could climb on it and slowly inch his way to the top of the pit and get out. The dirt rose so high that the donkey was able to climb right out of there! In the end, all those men shoveling dirt on the donkey helped it get out of the pit! The donkey could have given up but instead decided to persevere.

Whether a person knows it or not, some of the people or situations hurting you the most may be helping you grow in Christ. In the midwest's fall season, trees demonstrate the importance of letting the dead parts go. When spring arrives, so does new growth. Meditate on this and attempt to let go of the things that no longer serve you. If you discover the signs that God has set out for you, you will have the power to break free from the protective mechanisms of old wounds. Comfort yourself with faith and embrace the positive transformation that is to come. After all, Albert Einstein says, "In the middle of every difficulty lies opportunity."

 Psalm 107:19-21 ~ So they cried out to the Lord in their distress, and God saved them from their desperate circumstances. God gave the order and healed them; he rescued them from their pit. Let them thank the Lord for his faithful love and his wondrous works for all people.

PERSPECTIVE UPON RETURN

When you're in a dark place, you sometimes tend to think you've been buried. Perhaps you've been planted. Bloom.

~ Unknown

It has been fantastic to be home for a few weeks, and I'm slowly gaining energy. I go back to the hospital on Monday, October 13, for a week-long round of chemo and plan on returning home Saturday, October 18. This phase will be different from the induction phase. Now, I am in the consolidation phase, which means that I am in remission, and we want to keep it that way. My last bone marrow biopsy and aspiration showed no signs of CANcer in my bone marrow, but my doctor wants to make sure there are no more CANcer cells in my bloodstream that the biopsy may have missed. Therefore, consolidation is the next step toward long-term wellness.

Here's how my week of chemo is supposed to progress from what my doctors have told me. Monday, I check into the hospital by 8:00 a.m. Then they prep me for chemotherapy treatments consisting of two rounds on Monday, Wednesday, and Friday, having Tuesday and Thursday off. The chemo will be at the highest dose level again, but the medical care team mentioned that this wouldn't be as bad as the induction phase, which is encouraging. Since I am feeling good right now, I dread going back to the hospital because I know the chemo will make me feel lousy and deplete my immune system again. Even with this struggle to come, I am doing my best to maintain positivity.

Royal Treatment

Upon arrival and check-in at the hospital this morning, I knew that a new PICC line needed to be inserted into my arm before we could begin IV treatments. Knowing what to expect this time around, I wasn't as nervous, but a small part of me was still anxious. Partially because the shot given to numb the inside of my upper right arm is painful, but also because of the pressure I feel from the long PICC line insertion. What makes me most nervous is that the line is pushed until it rests just above my heart. And with all that, once the PICC line has entered my body, the feeling leaves me in a constant uncomfortable state. I could sense that a foreign object was in my body, and I couldn't wait for it to come out.

This PICC line procedure has been less stressful than my first visit, though. Last time, I cried when the nurse was finishing up; it wasn't because I was in a lot of pain, but rather that I was terrified. The most stressful feeling is not knowing what to expect or how this new chemo cocktail would affect me. After all, everyone's body is different, and side effects can be triggered by anything. The first time I had the procedure, my mind kept replaying movie scenes of actors undergoing chemo treatments. They always had horrific results. And let me just say right now, I hate vomiting! But I am so thankful that there are a lot of medications nowadays that drastically reduce nausea and vomiting. Being aware of this helps to calm my nerves. Each round of chemo draws me closer to the finish line, and I know that I'll come out the champion!

The fight in me didn't just happen overnight. I have always pushed myself through challenges by putting forth my best effort. For as long as I can remember, I've had the drive to succeed in whatever came my way. I never considered myself to be 'hard core' competitive. However, when it came to having a friendly contest, you could count me one-hundred percent in! Of course, if I happened to be the one who prevailed, then that was just icing on the cake.

When I was fifteen, my family traveled to Michigan for a Chevrolet Nomad Association Convention (classic cars). We only attended the convention for two or three years, but my recollections of these trips will always be dear to me. Back then, there were always activities for kids to participate in while the adults had their fun. The car association had an assortment of games, including those with small prizes for the top three winners.

One game, in particular, was a jump roping contest to see who could skip the most without stopping. It seemed like a fun and easy task, so I thought I'd give it a shot. Kids of all ages participated in this event. Some accomplished ten skips, while others completed seventy-two. When it was my turn, I began like any other contender, but I competed with my eye on the prize. The judge counted my skips – one hundred fifty-six... five hundred ninety-two... seven hundred ninety-eight. People started to gather around and count along with the judge. The crowd was amazed that I had been jumping for so long. Eventually, my feet tripped over the jump rope after reaching eight hundred ninety-two skips. I was awarded the first-place prize in this competition and still have it collecting dust in the back of my kitchen cabinet to this day – a pink Bart Simpson plastic cup.

From time to time, Bart's cup peaks through the shadows and provides the perfect opportunity to tell my kids the story behind this trophy of mine. Yes, the physical award was minimal, but my emotional and mental reward was through the roof! I was very proud of myself for putting forth my best effort and having it pay off. People I didn't even know congratulated me for days following the event.

Later that year, my parents received the quarterly Chevrolet Nomad Association Magazine in the mail and found a lovely surprise inside. There was a picture of me jumping rope and a brief description of the number of skips executed, titled *Jump Roping Queen!* It sure felt good to be recognized as a queen for my victory. A while back, my mom showed me the original copy of that magazine she saved all these years and is still delighted. I just smiled, remembering the feeling I had as a champion. I hadn't realized that it made my parents proud as well. Sometimes we all need a pat on the back for our accomplishments – no matter how big or small they are – to lift our spirits and give us an extra push to keep moving forward with the motivation of success.

1 Thessalonians 5:11 ~ Therefore encourage one another and build each other up, just as in fact you are doing.

A Day at Work

Today, I went for several walks in the hospital hallway to get the chemo moving through my system faster. While making the rounds, I met some great people. It's always nice to visit with patients going through similar situations. We lift each other's spirits, offer support, and reassure one another that we are not alone. It's good for us to share both the difficult and the easy times together. I also love seeing and visiting with the nurses. I honestly feel like the faculty and I have more than just a patient-provider relationship. The deep conversations we shared during my long-term stay in the hospital formed a bond unlike any other. I consider them my allies and familiars when I'm here.

As the day went on, my nurse came to my room to check on me. She was holding a fake ID badge with my picture on it and the words "G.I. Mary Jane," nurse at Methodist. She said, "I made this so I could put you to work and help your day go faster." I was pleasantly surprised that she cared enough to make my day magical.

This particular nurse gave such a warm welcome upon my initial arrival at the hospital when I was so scared. She was supportive and offered comfort when I broke down or asked many questions (because that's the way I am programmed). I'll never know exactly why my nurse did this for me or if this was something that was done for other patients in the past. I felt like I was important and genuinely meant something to her. It was then that I knew I wasn't alone in this fight.

Immediately after putting on the ID badge, we voyaged out of my hospital room to complete our mission – together. We took several pictures of me pretending to work and had some great laughs. I pushed a cart down the hall and checked another staff member's temperature and blood pressure. I faked answering the phone, welcoming guests, and typing on the receptionists' computer. All of this was such an incredible mood boost, as I had been fatigued all day. At the end of our adventure, I happily returned to my room and placed my fake ID badge on the counter next to family photos and the G.I. Mary Jane banner hanging on the wall. We all need to have some purpose to keep that spark alive inside us.

Speaking of, a spark can ignite from even the tiniest seeds of encouragement. For instance, I had another surprise experience that gassed up my flame the following day. My friend and mentor in the field of visual impairments stopped by for a visit. She has always been an inspiration, and I am glad we met a few years ago at a conference. This friend also happened to be a patient at Methodist (except on a different floor – for another reason). She took the risk of sneaking out of her room and boarding the elevator to pay me a visit. She arrived with a homemade door-hanging sign. It was a rubber glove with its fingers set in the shape of a 'rock on' sign, stuffed with none other than *Depends* underwear. The middle and ring fingers were folded down with tape, and a rubber band was attached underneath them for hanging purposes. The upright fingers represent the universal sign for "I love you." Only this particular friend would think of such a creation, and I felt so special knowing she had made it just for me. She hung the stuffed hand on the outside of my door, and I noticed she had drawn a heart and wrote "G.I. Mary Jane" on the front. She certainly put a bright spot in my day and helped me forget about the crumminess of cancer for a little while.

 Galatians 6:10 ~ Therefore, as we have opportunity, let us do good to all people, especially to those who belong to the family of believers.

PAY CLOSE ATTENTION TO THE SIGNS

The universe is always speaking to us...
sending us little messages, causing coincidences and serendipities,
reminding us to stop, to look around,
to believe in something else, something more.

~ Nancy Thayer

Shortly after I woke up on October 17, I became upset because my doctor told me that he planned to have my second round of chemo (in the consolidation phase) in four weeks instead of six. We discussed that the more chemo treatments I am able to tolerate, the better the outcome. If my body can handle it, he would like me to have three more rounds, set four weeks apart from this time on. Yes, I have to admit, I had a little 'feel sorry for myself' moment. I don't feel so hot right now and was hoping to have more time to recuperate before my next round of treatments began. I'm sure we have all gone through self-pity at one time or another. And I think it's healthy to take a step back and go through the motions in small doses, but also not let sadness or discouragement take over your life.

As the morning drew to a close, my nurse came into my room to hook my chemo bag onto the roll cart, and it happened... a few tears fell. I tried to stop them from streaming down my cheeks, but that just made the build-up of my emotional storm worse, and I began to sob. As Carl Jung said, "What you resist persists" so we must find a way to recover from the rumble caused by the boom.

My nurse showed compassion and told me to let it out if that's what I needed. So, that's what I did. It only lasted for a few minutes because crying is not something I like to do in front of others. It makes me feel inferior and vulnerable. I felt a lot better after doing so, though. I needed a release, some time for a pause, and a small break from this fight for life. It's necessary to sacrifice comfortability now and then when you're working towards your highest self. Shortly after my emotional breakdown began, I picked myself up and wiped the tears. I then ate my breakfast in peace, thanking God for this blessed day. After all, I'm in remission and still alive. Besides, I'm growing stronger in faith and courage with every step. There are always things to be grateful for in life. I just need to take a moment and watch for them.

Fortunately, it seems like there is always something happening in the hallway to make the time go by faster, so I decided to go for another stroll once I finished breakfast. After a few laps of my usual route, I ran into a friendly woman I met briefly a couple of days ago. We began talking, and she told me that I looked familiar to her (I felt the same). As we conversed further, we realized her daughter (another patient) was best friends with my cousin's wife, who passed away a few years ago. I went to her daughter's room to meet her. It was delightful! You just never know who you will bump into.

My heart was touched today when I visited with this woman and her ever-so-strong daughter. Ironically, as I write this, the song played at my cousin's funeral is now playing on the radio, called "Come to Jesus" by Chris Rice. God is among us all the time, masterminding every moment. I will never give up hope. I even sense that those who have passed on are standing strong with me in this battle. Perhaps, my late cousin wanted to give me this sign to let me know that she is with me.

 John 4:48 ~ "Unless you people see signs and wonders," Jesus told him, "you will never believe."

All in a Week

The brain is such a complex and wondrous organ. This past week has been quite a challenge... my mind had fixated on the positive feelings of remission and forgot about the not-so-good technicalities of the healing process after chemo. When I got home from the hospital, the first few days were mostly spent on the couch, watching movies, or napping. I had no energy, was nauseated, and my entire body ached terribly. Shaylee sat beside me often, and I could tell she craved big hugs. I had to remind her to be extra gentle because my skin hurt (as I put it). I find it interesting that my mind lets me forget that every fiber of my being is in pain during the recovery phase. I speculate that the chemo infuses into the muscles and organs, including the skin, to destroy all cells. This hypothesis is a bit dramatic, but it would explain why my body has been in so much pain for the past few days. It could also be from the shot implanted in my stomach to boost my white blood cells after each chemo round. I suppose the reason doesn't really matter. All I know is that my experience hasn't been fun.

After going through the chemo process more than once, I tend to go in thinking I know what will come next and have a sense of how my body will react. Unfortunately, my predictions are almost always false. Each of my recovery phases has come with its own unpredictable twists. This week, my eyes began hurting immensely. I have never felt so much pain in them before. I was prescribed steroid eye drops this time around to prevent retinal damage from the chemo and have been putting two drops in my eyes four times a day, as directed by my doctor. He told me to continue using the eye drops at home over the next week.

I didn't even think that the chemo could reach my eyes. Monday was the first real problematic day in my recovery. My eyes hurt terribly, and over the next few days, they didn't seem to feel any better no matter what I did. I even resorted to putting a patch over my right eye for nearly two days because that eye hurt the worst – even when closed. Bright lights, computer screens, TV, reading, and anything else I commonly used my vision for were especially harmful. Honestly, it felt like my cornea had been ripped open. Every time I blinked, the surface of my eye stung from the irritation. During my lab appointment on Monday, I asked the nurse about it, and she told me that the chemo just had to run its course. This news was very discouraging to hear, but I'm a fighter and will not let things like this break me, not even this intense eye pain.

My situation made me think of my students with visual impairments and the non-visual alternatives that they utilize to stay safe while traveling in their environment. Fortunately, I already had some of these skills in my survival toolbox and could put them to good use while I recovered. Yes, my temporary eye condition was very frustrating, but it also shifted my perception a bit. A few of my students have to be responsible for taking daily eye drops (for life) to preserve the limited vision they have left. For some, this causes discomfort or irritation when administered. They also needed to learn essential safety skills to prepare for independence. For all these years, I had taken my vision for granted because it was something that I always possessed freely. It is only now that I realize how much the quality of our sight can impact our livelihoods.

I am doing my best to see, with great clarity, what is essential in life. Everyone has their own views, attitudes, and vices, to name a few. My viewpoint regarding life has changed since discovering this illness. I departed from the hospital with a fresh set of lenses and immediately recognized how different I had become. My former way of life was to grab my kids from the bus stop, arrive at home, and have them start on homework as I rushed to prepare supper, eat, and clean up the kitchen. Afterward, I reminded my kids to shower and brush their teeth before putting them to bed and doing it all over again the next day.

Living in such a strained manner was unhealthy. I now know that time is valuable, and simplicity is appreciated. My worth is not defined through outward appearance or lists of accomplishments. At any given moment,

I have the power to proclaim a different ending to my story. There is no longer doubt or stress in my heart.

 James 1:2-4 ~ Consider it pure joy, my brothers and sisters, whenever you face trials of many kinds, because you know that the testing of your faith produces perseverance. Let perseverance finish its work so that you may be mature and complete, not lacking anything.

CHOOSE SOMETHING SWEET

*The key to being happy is knowing that you have
the power to choose what to accept and what to let go.*

~ Dodinsky

Most have heard the quote, "When life throws you lemons, make lemonade!" As manageable as that sounds, it's not always easy to recognize sweet twists when something sour comes at you full blast. It could be a sour attitude, sour expression, or a sour aura. If something leaves you feeling drained or upset, what's the point in trying to lighten it up? How is it even possible? The answer that comes to my mind is that it's only possible if you're willing to put in the effort.

Every day, I have a choice to wake up on the right or wrong side of the bed. My outlook in the morning will affect my decisions as the day progresses, just as how I treat others will affect *their* outlooks. It's a butterfly effect of kindness, so to speak. If someone tries to ruin my good mood, I now try to respond with nothing but LOVE. There is no need for petty digs at each other, and I'm no longer concerned with the idea of 'getting even.'

Thankfully, we have the God-given right of free will. We have the ability to check ourselves and listen to each other. Again, these days, I choose HOPE and LOVE. No matter how grim or despairing it may seem at times, everyone has a hope-filled future. It's never too late for a happily-ever-after. Keep praying for whatever 'joy' would lift you up the most. Create your best life by manifesting your dreams and desires like a magnet, drawing them towards you until they become a reality. I like to do this through prayer.

God hears our calls and often answers them in unexpected ways. Assistance might materialize in forms that we don't understand at first, but they will always follow through in the end – just like Cinderella's glass slipper.

Cinderella never asked her fairy godmother for a prince. She asked for a night off and a beautiful gown! Who knew that one evening and a pair of delicate shoes could change a life? Some things happen in the most miraculous of ways. As the saying goes, "If the shoe fits, wear it!" Life presents us with a multitude of shoes. Some don't fit quite right, others we grow out of, and most end up ruined from too much wear. Only a rare selection of shoes fit perfectly. We have a choice to either go through life with blisters from squeezing into the wrong footwear or to accept the gift of God's glass slipper. Don't pass up the opportunity to start leaving behind the right footprints.

Of course, I am fully aware that perfection is just an illusion. But what if something is perfect to *you* only? It may not seem perfect on the outside, but it may be just what you need in your life for some reason. After all, everyone has their own perception of what 'perfect' means to them. One person may regard something as perfect, while another looks at it like garbage. For instance, it has been about one month since I noticed the blisters on my feet were nearly healed from wearing high-heels. Now my feet look perfect – at least in my eyes. I chuckle at the thought of my 'funny' pinky toe that Tim teases me about now and then. The inherited fifth digit of a short stub sticking out of my foot with the smallest toenail seen by humankind. The nail even has a tiny ripple on one edge. It's definitely unique and used to be one of my insecurities. When my children were born, I checked their toes to see if they had a pinky toe like mine. Only one of my four kids inherited this generational trait. My short toe and funny nail may not seem perfect to others (if they look close enough to notice), but it's absolutely ideal for me. Regardless of how my little toe looks on the outside, it's a great way to remember my ancestors.

Thinking about all of this brings up the sweet topic of HOPE again. When I was first diagnosed with leukemia, I never gave up hope. Even though this news destroyed the 'perfect' image of my life, it allowed me to focus on what was important – my health and happiness. Hope was something that I could hold onto, keeping my spirits up when times were tough during treatment. I found that concentrating on favorable outcomes helped me tackle unpleasant situations. Sometimes it is hard for us to understand the purpose of pain. Why did God choose to put me through these trials? Did I bring this suffering upon myself? I can only hope that CANcer points me towards answers and teaches me how to prioritize the things that actually matter.

We can all use a reminder about the possibility of happy endings. Let's remember that Jesus died for us on the cross, giving us the freedom of choice. Don't take this freedom for granted. Go ahead and make some lemonade out of your lemons! Or bake a cake with the dusty ingredients in your cupboard! Trust me, I wish that I had followed my heart when I had the chance. Right now, I'm just sitting in my bed praying for another opportunity. Don't let the diet of conformity hold you back from your sweet passions. Always choose what you most enjoy.

 Hebrews 6:19 ~ This hope is a strong and trustworthy anchor for our souls. It leads us through the curtain into God's inner sanctuary.

ALLOWING THE RAIN TO WASH ME CLEAN

Even the stones placed in one's path
can be made into something beautiful.

~ Wolfgang Goethe

On Wednesday, November 7, Tim drove me to Estabrook for labs and an appointment. My doctor informed me that my numbers are high enough to receive the second round of chemo in the consolidation phase. I will be at the hospital from November 10-15. I'm not sure my mind is ready for the next round, but my doctor said it's best to stay on schedule. We need to make sure that any lingering cancer cells are destroyed. Just like healthy cells, cancer cells have the ability to recover. This means that we need to knock them down before they have any chances of recuperating and multiplying. Each round of chemo will be harder on my body and may take longer for me to bounce back from, but research proves that four one-week-long rounds of chemo are ideal for long-term remission and cure.

As I sat with this information longer, it hit me hard. I told my doctor that I dreaded going back for another round. I am just beginning to feel better but am still fatigued. The tears started to fall, and I couldn't stop them. I apologized and told him that I usually don't get this upset, especially not in front of him. He said not to fret and that I was handling this situation well. I think I was so emotional because I know what chemo does to my body, and it's not a pleasant experience. It would be nice to wait a little longer, but I know what I have to do.

Tim drove us home, and it was quiet. Then he reminded me of all the great things my doctor said about how I was doing. It's funny, I didn't remember most of the good comments. Sometimes it's easier to think about the negative, even when so many great things are happening around us. I'm so glad Tim was with me for this appointment. It's always a good idea to have a loved one with you when receiving a lot of information to ensure that it ALL gets heard.

Shortly after we got home, I left to get the kids from the bus stop. I was almost down my lane when the rain started to hit my vehicle with great force. It came out of nowhere! I looked toward the sky and only saw a couple spots with dark storm clouds. The majority of the sky was brightly lit by the sun, with a few scattered fluffy white clouds. I kept driving, and the rain began to pound more fiercely on my vehicle as if it was trying to get my attention. I had this overwhelming feeling of calmness and cleansing come over me as if the rain was washing me clean. I reached the highway and noticed that the rain had stopped abruptly. My children arrived at the bus stop shortly after me, and we went to my parents' house for a short while. I told them that it was raining hard by my house and noticed their place was bone dry (they live about five miles from me). My parents thought that was strange because it didn't look like it was going to rain at their house at all. I didn't think much more of it until last night. My friend, who lives about two miles from me, texted a message along with a picture. She wrote, "Did you see the rainbow yesterday?" Wow, God is so good! I know He was sending a message. Maybe something like, "Hey, I got this, no need to be disheartened! It's a good day!"

I continue to pray that all will go according to God's plan, and I return home safely after chemo next week. Interesting observation: After the induction phase, I was scheduled to go home on my wedding anniversary.

Following the first round in the consolidation phase, I was able to go home on my dad's birthday. And upon completing this next round of chemo, I will return home on my daughter Holly's birthday on November 15. Isn't that fascinating? What are the odds?

It occurred to me that all of these dates hold a special meaning in my heart and are more signs from God. I began to notice the significance of this pattern. I realized that every time I came home from a temporary stay in the hospital, there had also been a celebration of life within my family. I understand that these celebrations don't necessarily relate to *my* life. Still, the meaning behind these occasions brings forth a 'feel good' emotion that sends positive endorphins throughout my body to aid in the healing process.

These important family events only happen once a year, and it just so happens that they have occurred on each day that I've come home from another round of chemo. What's even crazier is that my chemo treatments give me LIFE, and I return home on these celebrations of LIFE. God makes connections like this everywhere. Finding His personal touches makes overcoming my struggles that much easier. Search for His messages in your life.

 2 Corinthians 5:7 ~ For we live by faith, not by sight.

Coincidence, I think NOT!

The morning arrived for me to return to the hospital for the second round of chemo. Before I knew it, my dad was at my house to drive me to the hospital since Tim was working out of town. When we got there, the receptionist checked me in. She picked up the phone and said, "Mary Robinson is ready to go upstairs to room 602." I perked right up and told her that #602 was my favorite room! I was so excited to get THAT room! What are the odds of that? Once again, God was letting me know that He was with me. My first stay in room 602 was during my recovery from the induction phase. While there, I found out I was in remission and had two miracles. Plus, the shower is much warmer. The beautiful view of the trees outside that window also reminds me of the scenery at my house. When we arrived at room 602, I felt right at home. There were a lot of familiar faces, all of which have always been friendly and welcoming.

After settling in, I was given steroids and nausea medication through an IV to prepare for chemo. Then one of the nurses set up the chemo bag on the IV cart. The other nurse asked me what radio station I was listening to, which happened to be a local Christian radio station. I told her that I have it playing twenty-four hours a day while in the hospital. Then she began telling me some inspirational stories about how God has been there for her. It's always encouraging to hear about how God works in the lives of others. When people tell their uplifting stories, it further confirms our own magical experiences. These are real signs that the universe works in our favor.

To give me a sense of peace, I regularly sit by a window in my hospital room and gaze up to the sky. Recently, I've been noticing rainbows more often than ever before. Their frequent appearances got me thinking about the dove that Noah released after the great flood. He asked the dove to return with an olive branch to find out if there was dry land (written in the book of Genesis). God promised Noah that He would never flood the Earth again, and this covenant was sealed with the promise of a rainbow. I think this promise has resonated with me for my entire life.

When I was much younger, I would catch myself in daydreams, searching for figures in the clouds. I loved watching the white fluffs morph into new shapes and drift away. There is something about the calming effect that radiates from a blue sky. I often wondered if a person could just bounce from one cloud to another, frolicking with pure freedom. I imagined the clouds as a sort of 'heaven on earth,' like they were just giant marshmallows holding the souls of our deceased loved ones. These 'marshmallow homes' in the sky were places of majestic wonder, love, and hope. My young self knew that I would be reunited with my family after death.

Back to my room in the hospital, the clouds continued to float off to nowhere. Suddenly, I spotted a beautiful rainbow peeking out between the hazy sky-puffs. Would you look at that? For most, rainbows show up when they're least expected. But in my case, the bright colors poke through when I need them most.

 Romans 8:28 ~ And we know that in all things God works for the good of those who love him, who have been called according to his purpose.

BEAUTIFUL TESTIMONY OF FAITH

Faith allows things to happen.
It is the power that comes from a fearless heart.
And when a fearless heart believes, miracles happen.

~ Unknown

Oh, the power of prayer! God works quickly if we ask and wait with a patient heart. I am having a great day, and I refuse to let anything knock me off of this feeling. Thank goodness I have so many praying for me. This morning, my doctor came into my room and couldn't believe that my blood counts looked so good. All the numbers miraculously went up, and I am no longer in isolation. Since we had no explanation, I attribute it to the power of prayer and my good mood!

After the excellent news, I found myself captivated by a distant memory from March 2011 when I went to a Women's Christian retreat in Colorado. Attending the retreat was a new experience for me, so I wasn't sure what to expect. Initially, I went to recharge and rejuvenate, but God brought some unexpected reflections to the surface. During the retreat, there was a session on "What is your given name?" Names are significant, and I believe these titles end up meshing perfectly with each individual's personality as they blossom into adulthood.

As a child of God, Jesus has a name for all of us. I'm not talking about the birth name given to you by your parents or caregivers. From what I remember, our 'other' name could be something like "Courageous," "Beloved," or "Strong." Sometimes, Jesus gives a person more than one name. Other times, an individual could be given a part of scripture or quote as a name. It varies from person to person. At the end of this particular session, we had the opportunity to walk to the front of the room to grab a white rock and a sharpie pen to write our given names on the rock.

In that moment of quiet time and prayer, I asked Jesus to tell me my given name. At first, I was nervous because I looked around and noticed that some women were already at the front of the room claiming their rock. I thought, "What is their name, and how did they discover it so quickly?" There I went again, worrying about what was going on around me instead of focusing on my own task. I chose to close my eyes and continue to pray.

It came to me just like that; I heard "Faith." At first, I thought, "Faith? Could that be right? It seems too simple." I wondered if I had just conjured that up in my head. But I wrote the name "Faith" on my new rock anyway and went about the day. Toward the evening, we were settling down to sleep, and I asked Jesus to confirm my given name one more time. I heard it loud and clear, "Faith!"

Fast forward to yesterday, I received a gift from the couple in the hospital, whom I now consider friends. Inside a little box was a heart-shaped rock with the word "Faith" engraved on one side. I held onto it with pride and trust. To me, this is a sacred reminder to keep the faith during times of trials and tribulations. It also took me back to that memory at the retreat a few years ago. It was as if God was poking me in the side to alert me of my true identity. He was saying, "You ARE Faith, Mary. I am with you always." As my grip tightened around the rock of faith, I pondered over this hard truth and came to realize that this simple five-letter word – FAITH – is more substantial and of greater value than most can grasp. Faith has the potential to be combined with many layers of hope if we allow it. In fact, without the symbolic partnership with faith, what else do we have? I believe the answer is: Nothing.

Towards the end of that same retreat, I remember hearing a song that spoke to me, and I closed my eyes. I had a vision of myself floating in a glorious scene of a lush forest. My body was wrapped in a long white garment, and I floated with my head and arms tilted back. I felt extreme peace in every cell of my body and had a closed-mouth smile on my face. As I slowly rose off the ground, my body began to spin ever so slowly. It was in that moment that I felt renewed and cleansed from all my sins. It was an incredible experience – one that I will never forget. And I think that's the whole point. It's not always easy, but in moments of trial, it's our job to remember who we are and who is holding us dear all the time.

 2 Corinthians 4:18 ~ So we fix our eyes not on what is seen, but on what is unseen since what is seen is temporary, but what is unseen is eternal.

THE GOOD LIFE

Every day may not be good,
but there is something good in every day.

~ Alice Morse Earle

For as long as I can remember, the state of Nebraska's trademark has always been "The Good Life." Yes, I believe Nebraska is a pleasant place to live, but I have always wondered how this state got its slogan. So, I researched a bit and found that "The Good Life" is Nebraska's original state slogan. In the 1970s, an advertising firm from Omaha created it at the governor's request. Since then, there have been fourteen different slogans in Nebraska. I suppose "The Good Life" catchphrase is not going away anytime soon because they keep going back to it.

The other day I was thinking about what a good life means to me. It's not all about materialistic items, fame, or fortune, although those things sure sound delightful. Or do they? What's the price of fame or fortune? When a person has the drive to give up so much to reach the top, it raises the question: "Is it all worth it?" Honestly, I don't know; it depends on the situation.

We all have the power to gauge the weight of our sacrifices as we pursue goals. And it will often be that our judgment is misguided. For some, I think it's all about the climb, adrenaline rush, or thrill of what it takes to get to their destination. A few also have higher aspirations ingrained in their DNA and will do whatever it takes to succeed. When individuals work hard to rise above, they feel satisfaction from the reward of accomplishments. Unfortunately, this is a good way to isolate yourself and destroy relationships with those who care about you. Mistreating others on your way to success is a sacrifice that will never be worth it.

In contrast to the high-strung type-A personalities, there are the more relaxed, go-with-the-flow type-Bs. This group tends to have more laid-back dispositions and take the easier route. They seize the day and focus on simple pleasures in life. Type-Bs are content with navigating through daily tasks without the physical and mental pressure of advancement. Both walks of life have their advantages. However, since I've primarily been in the type-A category for most of my adult life, I'm growing weary of my high expectations to continue in this rat race. My illness forced me to slow down and gave me a chance to realize the only thing that matters: FAMILY.

My perspective has changed drastically since going through the drama of recovery. To me, a good life is about spending quality time with loved ones and building lifelong memories. It's about nurturing my soul, staying grounded, and practicing an attitude of gratitude. I've learned that finding the right balance of work and leisure is also a key component to maintaining overall happiness. Additionally, a monumental achievement of mine has been learning to trust whatever outcome presents itself. Regardless of what I may think is best or suitable at the moment, I have learned to lean into faith, knowing that God has control over every situation. CANcer knocked down the branches of my tree, and I never thought anything positive would come from that. But, in retrospect, the mushrooms of blessings have sprouted from those dead limbs. I can't wait to harvest these new growths.

Frankly, it doesn't matter what state a person lives in or whether they are a cruiser or an over-achiever. Everyone's experiences are different, but here's one thing that is consistent for all: Companionship is the only way for us to evolve. Reflections of our accomplishments lose weight when the mirrors break and we realize we're all alone.

My children are growing so fast, and before I know it, they will graduate from high school and move on with their life. I want to have a solid relationship with my kids while they still live with me and be a positive role model as they mature into adulthood. It's never too late to make a fresh start. Take a pause and think about how you can boost these connections.

A song came to my mind while writing this. It's called "He Knows My Name" by Francesca Battistelli. This tune reminds me that no matter how we lead our lives or what career path we take, God knows our name. That's what *really* matters. Be true to who you are. You are famous in God's eyes!

Interestingly enough, recently, I needed to renew my driver's license. A short time after, I received my license in the mail. Inside the envelope (in big letters), I read, "Nebraska, Good Life. Great Future." Ahh, I love the sound of that. Yes, it is a good life, and I know it will be a fantastic future! Well said, and a perfect add-on to the original slogan.

 Psalm 119:105 ~ Your word is a lamp for my feet, a light on my path.

THE VOICE INSIDE MY HEAD

*The value of persistent prayer is not that He will hear us
but that we will finally hear Him.*

~ William McGill

It's December 8, and I can't believe it's already time for me to return to the hospital for another round of chemo. It seems as if time has been working double shifts during this recovery phase. I woke up in the middle of the night with a lot on my mind. As I was lying in bed, all of a sudden I heard, "Your faith has made you well." I immediately opened my eyes and looked around my dark, silent room. I saw nothing out of the ordinary. Then, with newfound peace, I closed my eyes and thanked God for all His blessings.

That incident reminded me of a Bible scripture in the book of Matthew. There was a woman who had been suffering from hemorrhaging for several years. She had sought help and endured a great deal under the care of many doctors, but no one could stop the bleeding. In fact, she was getting worse, and no longer had money to seek help. This woman heard about Jesus and believed she would be healed if she could just touch His clothing. Now that's what I call FAITH! Matthew 9:20-22 states, "Just then a woman who had been subject to bleeding for twelve years came up behind Him [Jesus] and touched the edge of his cloak. She said to herself, 'If I only touch his cloak, I will be healed.' Jesus turned and saw her. 'Take heart, daughter,' he said, 'your faith has healed you.' And the woman was healed at that moment."

Jesus performed many miracles during His life on Earth and continues to execute them today. I firmly believe that I will beat this, just as the woman in the Bible story overcame her illness. God continues to hold my hand as I work my way around this stretch of obstacles. I am so grateful for His consistency and will rest easy knowing that my faith is making me well.

 John 16:33 ~ "I have told you these things, so that in me you may have peace. In this world you will have trouble. But take heart! I have overcome the world."

FAMILY TAKES CARE OF FAMILY

Other things may change us, but we start and end with family.

~ Anthony Brandt

My dad picked me up from the hospital on Saturday, December 13. This past week went faster than usual, and I am very grateful. It is always incredible to get home after an extended stay at the hospital and see my children and husband. I am welcomed with a first-rate attitude each time. The house is consistently clean. The kids are always thoughtful and ask if I need anything throughout the day. I can just sit, relax, and heal – at least most of the time.

Christmas seemed to be approaching rapidly this year. Fortunately, Holly, Colby, and Shaylee wanted to decorate the tree by themselves during Thanksgiving break. They did such a fabulous job! Honestly, the tree looks better this year than all the previous years when I set it up myself. Even though I am still struggling from a lack of energy, I am super excited to spend quality time with family during the Christmas holiday. However, this Christmas will look slightly different because I often go in for labs and blood transfusions.

On Saturday, December 20, Shaylee came to me when she woke up and started crying excessively. I asked her what was wrong, and she said that she had a cold. I felt terrible for her because she was worried about my health, with little regard to hers. I assured her that she couldn't help it if she got a cold and that we would get through this.

Brody had a birthday party that same day, but thankfully, we didn't plan for it to be at our house. He chose to go to the movies with his friends. Tim and Matt were very willing to help. I knew they could handle Brody's birthday party, so I sent them off with the cake and party favors. The celebration went great with Tim and Matt in charge. I stayed at home with Shaylee, being extra cautious while tending to her needs from a comfortable distance. My intentions were to give Shaylee a feeling of security about my health remaining intact because she genuinely was concerned about my wellbeing. I didn't want her to feel guilty about getting sick because it was not her fault and could have happened to anyone in the family. Her job was to get better, not to worry about me.

As the morning went on, I checked her temperature because she was not very active…102.8 degrees – YIKES! I was a little anxious (okay, maybe extremely nervous), but I tried my best not to show it. My white blood count was at 200. The normal range is 4,500-11,000 mcL, and my numbers were not expected to rise for quite some time. I got a shot in my torso six days ago to help reboot my white blood cells faster, but it takes up to ten days to begin working. In other words, it was still a critical time for me to maintain wellness. I called my mom, and she had the best advice – wear a mask. So, I did just that! To ease Shaylee's mind, I told her that I was going to cover my face with a mask and disinfect the house while wearing disposable gloves. Shaylee was such a trooper and did her best to stay on the couch in an effort not to spread germs any further. I gave her medicine to keep the fever from spiking too high and placed a cool washcloth on her forehead, but I was not able to cradle her or soothe her in my arms as I had in the past. Shaylee didn't complain, though. She must have understood why it had to be this way.

Tinsel in a Tangle

Children are the anchors that hold a mother to life.

~ Sophocles

Sunday morning came, and I checked Shaylee's temperature when she woke up – it was 103.5 degrees! I immediately drew a bath and gave her more medicine. Fortunately, Shaylee was showing some life and was not entirely miserable. Tim and I decided that it would be best if he and Shaylee stayed at our family cabin for a couple of days so I wouldn't be exposed more than I already had been. I was relieved that Tim felt comfortable with the responsibilities of taking care of a sick child on his own. I knew that Shaylee was in good hands with her father. After they left, I sprayed disinfectant everywhere. We kept in touch by phone for the next two days, and Tim always gave me a recount of their time together. They watched a few movies, and he did his best to keep her spirits up as she recovered without having me by her side.

Since Tim was with Shaylee, my dad drove me to Omaha for labs on Monday morning. We found out that my hemoglobin was low, and I needed two units of blood. It was too late for the infusion center to take me because we needed to wait for my cross-matching blood results (testing done before every blood transfusion to determine if the donor's blood is compatible with the recipient's blood). This technicality meant that I needed to receive my transfusion at the hospital instead.

Unfortunately, this procedure takes much longer at the hospital because they have to provide care for the *entire* hospital, whereas the infusion center only has to provide for their patients. I can't complain, though. No matter the place, the staff takes such good care of us. My dad didn't grumble once and stayed with me all day until we got home around 7:00 p.m. I'm also so glad my mom was with the other three kids because it would have been such a long day for them to be home alone.

Shaylee and Tim came home on Tuesday morning (even though Shaylee still had a fever of 100.8 degrees) because Tim had a business meeting. I wore a mask and frequently sanitized, doing my best to reduce exposure. Shaylee felt much better than before and was very cooperative with me, which helped ease my anxiety. It must have been difficult for Shaylee, at her young age, to understand the precautions we were taking. And perhaps she even wondered if things were always going to be this way from now on. As a mother, I wanted nothing more than to be with her while she got over this terrible cold. I felt like I let her down by being too worried about my own health, even though I knew I needed to take these precautions. Regardless, all that really mattered was that we made it through another obstacle.

On Wednesday, Shaylee woke up without a fever. Tim and I were so relieved! I still wore a mask that day in case her fever came back and continued to pray for good health. Only one more week of chemo in January, and then I'm done for good. I can't wait until it's all over and everything gets back to normal – whatever that is anymore.

Tim's mother, Vickie, drove from western Nebraska to join us for Christmas. Unfortunately, his sister couldn't come because her girls were sick. I was worried enough about Shaylee's illness, and I just couldn't risk being in contact with another ailment if at all possible. Thank goodness they all understood.

Matt's three kids (ages sixteen, thirteen, and nine) came to visit from Arizona during the week of Christmas. It was great having them here since we don't get to see them very often. It brought some normalcy to the holiday, which was quite the refreshment after my hectic time in the hospital. All the cousins get along wonderfully and make lifelong memories with each visit. I've always felt it was necessary for them to get to know each other before adulthood. In my opinion, having a tight-knit family is vital. I will never take the most important people in my life for granted.

These days, my thoughts are often preoccupied with my family – not just my children and husband, but my parents and brother, too. My original family has always been close; that's why it's so important to me that my children have a strong bond with each other as well. My family story goes like this: I'd like to believe I had what most would call a typical childhood. We had a solid Christian upbringing and went to church nearly every Sunday. While growing up, I looked up to my older brother, Matt. I always knew that if things got tough, he would be there to listen and fervently watch out for me. I have always cherished our relationship and know that he's consistently had my best interest at heart.

When we were little, I was considered 'one of the boys' and frequently spent time with them. I guess you could call me a tomboy. I even have a few battle scars from accidental injuries while roughhousing over the years. Luckily, our mom was always there to bandage me up before the next escapade. We would invent new ways to play with leftover scraps lying on the ground from construction sites nearby, and our favorite pastime was riding our bikes so fast that we could let go of the handlebars and cruise! Matt and I were known to climb dirt mounds and play a *King of the Hill* game on many occasions. Fishing, swimming, and park adventures were also musts. We didn't seem to be afraid of anything because we always had each other's back.

Matt and I often ran across the street to the bowling alley from the convenient location of our house in Columbus. We got into the habit of foolishly spending our hard-earned money (what little we had) on arcade video games or the Claw Machine to capture a toy prize. We did nearly everything together with the neighborhood kids until we moved to western Nebraska.

Both of our lives were much different after our relocation. It was tough to have a sense of belonging in our new territory at the ages of eleven and thirteen. Life didn't seem so perfect anymore. We continued on our path by sticking together. Matt was there for me through emotional breakdowns from arguments with other girls, quarrels with our parents, or dramatic boyfriend breakups. We didn't hang out that much as we got older, but the bond between us could never be severed.

After Matt graduated high school and moved states away, I was still confident that I could always count on him. I want my children and their cousins to form a bond as strong as the one Matt and I have. It was clear that they had no chance of sharing adventures when they were separated by twelve hundred miles, so I took it upon myself to bring them together. Although it wasn't often, I can tell it made a difference, and I can only hope that they continue to maintain their relationships as they mature.

Over the years, Matt and I haven't visited as often as I'd like. Possibly because life doesn't stop moving, and we don't take the time to make a simple phone call just to say hello. Having said this, I never realized just how important the bond between my parents and brother was until I needed them most. It seems that these types of bonds, forged over time and built with a strong foundation, stay connected no matter the distance.

Shortly after Christmas, Matt's six-month stay in Nebraska came to an end. My health was moving in the right direction, so he thought it was time to move back to Arizona to spend more time with his children. Before Matt left, he gave me a big bear hug, filling me with the same sense of safety that I know so well, along with a soft kiss on the forehead. He then handed me a sealed envelope and stepped into his truck. When the door closed behind him, I quickly ran outside for one more goodbye wave, as I knew it would be many months until I saw him again.

Upon returning inside, I sat on the couch and opened the letter. It was as if I could hear Matt's voice speaking inside my head:

"Mary, you are such a strong and spiritual person. That's what I love about you. I know I don't normally write letters to you, but mom wouldn't let me have the phone whenever you called." I paused for a minute, chuckling because I could totally see my mom hogging the phone. Matt also adds so much humor to every situation, boosting people up with his wit and charm. I went on to read: "And as you know, mom likes to run the show. So I came up with a new name for her: *The General*. Ask Tim, dad, or me about it. Mom runs the shop around here. She is truly the backbone of this family, and I'm not sure I realized this until now, probably because I haven't been around you guys very often in the last several years. It was nice to be here for you these past six months. Anyway, if there is somebody stronger than you, Mary, it's mom. When I feel down and out, I look at mom, doing what she always does. She's a rock that never breaks. I say, 'Mom, you're going to wear yourself out!' She's always doing laundry, taking care of the grandkids, and helping with homework when you're in the hospital or recovering from treatments. I'm sure she helped a lot before all of this too. But, I guess that's the teacher in her. After I say that she's going to wear herself out (in a stern voice), she turns around and says to me, 'Matt, mind your own business! I'm fine, and I'll do what I want! Here in Nebraska, we stick together and help each other out. We're family, and family does what we need to do, so shut up!' There were a few more words than that too. I guess size doesn't matter. Look at mom – she's 4' 10," and we don't mess with her. I love mom so much! She's the strongest, kindest, most inspirational person I know. Mary, you have a lot of her genes in you. That's why I know you are going to be okay. I love you and will be a phone call away if you need anything. Love your favorite brother, Matt."

After reading the letter, I placed it near my heart and stared out the window for a few minutes. I noticed the limbs on the trees blowing in all directions from the cold, harsh December wind. I thought about the strength of a tree trunk and how it endures the seasonal changes, along with the strong winds that have been whipping it since the day it was planted. But the tree refuses to break, bend, or fall, for its roots are deep within the fertile soil. It's the struggle from years of bashing that gives the tree its beauty and its strength. Trees develop a resistance to the intense blows. I believe my family is like a tree. Our relationship can withstand any degree of weather. As I sat there, reflecting on Matt's note, I thought it was sure nice to have him close these past few months. After so many years of having over a thousand miles separating us, I felt like we reconnected. Instead of one of our week-long visits over the holiday once a year, I had the opportunity to get to know Matt (as an adult) on a more intimate level. I know that our bond will always withstand the test of time.

Furthermore, Matt is right; my mother is the rock and foundation of our family. I am so grateful for her strength. Both of my parents have helped me so much during each stage of recovery. I am so glad they moved within ten minutes from my house after retirement. Who knew that I would need my parents (more than ever) to get through it all? Dr. T. P. Chia says, "Parental love is the only love that is truly selfless, unconditional and forgiving." This quote is very accurate, in my case. I don't know what I would have done without the support of my parents. They are the best role models, not only for myself but also for the rest of my family. My kids know that we take care of each other in our family – regardless of the obstacles life throws at us. Together, we can get through anything.

 1 Peter 5:10 ~ And the God of all grace, who called you to his eternal glory in Christ, after you have suffered a little while, will himself restore you and make you strong, firm and steadfast.

Tick-Tock Goes the Clock

God didn't promise days without pain, laughter without sorrow, or sun without rain, but He did promise strength for the day, comfort for the tears, and light for the way. If God brings you to it, He will bring you through it.

~ Unknown

Monday, January 5, snuck up on me. Most likely because of the holidays. I am a little anxious just thinking about being in the hospital for chemo again, which has been the trend. So, I found myself crying once more. It is healthy to acknowledge these feelings of uncertainty, experience them, and then move on when I feel ready. I know that I need to complete all of these treatments to live a long-term life, but I am *very* over it. At least this is the final round of chemo.

I want to take this time to say how grateful I am to everyone at Methodist. The medical care team has been incredible – they make my stay the best it can be. Since I *have* to be experiencing this, it is comforting to know that the nurses, chaplain, and other staff members are willingly by my side. I will miss them when this is all over. They have been a tremendous support system.

When I arrived at the hospital and got settled into my room, I decided to go for a walk. Maybe seeing some familiar faces would lift my spirits. Each treatment has taken a toll on my body, and I'm not looking forward to going through side effects once again.

On Tuesday, I needed extra motivation to walk the halls. I was exhausted, somewhat nauseous, and didn't feel like drinking water or eating. Even so, I did my best not to complain. I am almost done fighting and look forward to letting my guard down. Tim continues to shower me with jokes and laughter. He also surprises me with food, hoping that something he provides will taste good.

Time is moving so quickly. It's already Thursday. When my doctor came to check on me this morning, he pointed out that I only had two treatments left. Wow, it's difficult to wrap my head around the fact that I'm almost done. Six months ago, my CANcer treatment to-do list looked like it would never end! I was also glad to hear that Matt didn't need to be tested for a stem cell transplant. The chemo was going to do the trick.

As I dove deeper into a daydream of prosperity, my nurse counselor walked in. We briefly visited, and I asked if there were any beneficial programs to improve my overall recovery. She talked to me about a program called *A Time to Heal*. This twelve-week session is designed to support men and women in regaining physical, emotional, intellectual, psychological, and spiritual health after undergoing cancer treatment. *A Time to Heal* promotes restorative health and is only a three-hour meeting, once a week. That doesn't sound too bad! Plus, I will get to meet new people. It might be encouraging to converse with other survivors and caregivers. This program sounds like a great way to emerge out of my CANcer journey.

As much as I will miss the staff at Methodist, I am ready to move on. I know that FAITH got me to the end of treatments, and I am HOPEFUL for the future. I realize that I may not be the same woman I was before this dreadful disease, but that's okay with me. I am looking forward to what *this* woman can accomplish with a new perspective, and I am SO grateful that I am almost done.

 Hebrews 13:15-16 ~ Through Jesus, therefore, let us continually offer to God a sacrifice of praise—the fruit of lips that openly profess his name. And do not forget to do good and to share with others, for with such sacrifices God is pleased.

HIT THE ROAD, MARY!

Home should be an anchor, a port in a storm, a refuge,
a happy place in which to dwell, a place where we are loved
and where we can love.

~ Marvin J. Ashton

It's Friday, January 9, 2015, and today has been full of mixed emotions. By midnight tonight, I will have met my goal and completed ALL rounds of chemotherapy in the consolidation phase. As I settle into the hospital chair, warm from the heat of the late afternoon sun, I take a moment to reflect on this day. It began with Tim arriving early this morning to spend time with me. Around noon, he noticed that I was having a difficult time finding something that sounded good to eat for lunch and decided to get me some food at a nearby restaurant. It was delicious – a nice change from the hospital menu. After a while, nothing had been sounding good to eat anymore, so I was grateful that Tim could find something to satisfy me for now. Don't get me wrong, the food at the hospital is lovely, and there are many options to choose from, but it's so inviting when I'm surprised with something different. I appreciate all that Tim does for me. I couldn't have asked for a better partner to stand alongside me in this challenge.

In addition to the lovely gesture from Tim, a volunteer cosmetologist also gave me a manicure. She stops by one to two times a month to make patients feel beautiful. The cosmetologists provide many color choices of nail polish, and we get to sit and relax while they work their magic. I chose an orange color to represent the leukemia ribbon. My nails haven't looked this fantastic in a long time! It always makes me feel pretty when I look down at my fingers and see a well-kept set of nails, especially when I'm not feeling so hot on the inside.

When Tim left to go home for the day, I decided to go for a short walk. I thought I heard my name but kept going. Then, it was louder and clearly voiced, "Mary!" I turned around and saw my nurse, who met me in the breezeway. She walked with me for a short while as we rounded the corner. Suddenly, many nurses and other staff surprised me with a delicious carrot cake while singing, "Hit the road, Mary! And don't you come back no more, no more! Hit the road, Mary, and don't you come back no more." I will never forget how much they cared about me and know my love for music so well. But how could they not know? Christian music has been playing in my room ALL the time. The nurses also must have *really* been listening when I mentioned my family's love for carrot cake months prior. What a generous medical care team I've had!

Wow, I hadn't realized that I had also made an impact on them these past six months. It was a moment of truth. I wasn't just a patient to them; I was a comrade who mattered. It was a 'happy' emotional time filled with laughter and many farewell hugs. Being discharged from the hospital is a joyous occasion, even though it means leaving behind the friends I've made in these halls. I can't imagine that the nurses do this kind of celebration for every patient, not to say that I am more special than others. Regardless, I believe we developed more than a patient and caregiver relationship. We shared stories, joys, fears, laughs, and even tears (on my end anyway). I felt so loved and accepted for being all that I am, leaving nothing concealed. The nurses gave G.I. Mary Jane the perfect marching orders: "Hit the road!" I will miss their company as I advance to new beginnings.

After all the excitement, it was pleasant to 'just be,' sedentary in the chair of my hospital room. I spent this quiet time thinking of how far I've come while gazing out the window. I would often catch glimpses of shimmering white snow falling from tree limbs after a big gust of wind. As I continued gazing off, a chill ran up my spine, and I tightly wrapped myself in the colorful blanket that my mother-in-law crocheted for me. In just a few short hours, I am leaving this room for good. Tomorrow, I will be home. As excited as I am, however, I cannot lie and say that I don't feel a bit of sadness to leave this place. The kind of love I felt here reminds me of how Jesus was to all humans when He walked on this earth. He did not judge, ridicule, or chastise. He did not boast, turn His cheek, or grumble. Instead, Jesus held out His gentle hand and helped those in need.

Compassion comes to mind as I write this, as it was at the forefront of my stay here. I wasn't alone in facing the challenges of healing, and the support of my team is the reason I'm here today. They never failed to swoop in and remind me why I was here. After all, positivity brings possibility. I needed to turn my focus inward to win the prize of life, and I WON. This valuable lesson showed me that I have what it takes to manifest desires beyond the imaginable. As Sonia Ricotti says matter of factly, "To live your greatest life, you must first become a leader within yourself. Take charge of your life, begin attracting and manifesting all that you desire in life." I did just that. And I take pleasure in reaping the ultimate reward: LIFE.

Tonight is my final round of chemo, and I get to go home tomorrow morning. When my nurse came to my room this evening, she surprised me with a colorful sign that read, "This is my final bag of chemo 4 ever!" Her encouraging message put me in the perfect mindset to finish strong. It's mind-boggling to be at the end of this long road. Now more than ever, I continue to declare: God is so good!

It was getting late, so I settled into bed. Before drifting off to sleep, I reread the note that the nurses handed me at my surprise celebration. It said: "Mary, we can't find the words to tell you how very happy we are for you in finishing up your chemo treatments. You have hung in there, remained strong with great courage and faith to get through it all. You truly are a special, one-of-a-kind lady, and I know the staff on 6 South are going to miss you too. You always have a way of lifting everyone else's spirits while going through treatments. Our prayers are for you and your family to now be able to get back to life as usual. Luv & Hugs."

The following day flew by. I went on my usual walk in the hallway in hopes of seeing my friends one last time before returning home. The excitement about my new beginning was hard to contain as I conversed with the nurses, other patients, and caregivers. I told everyone that I would stop by occasionally – especially since I needed to report back a few times a week for lab work, appointments, and blood transfusions next door.

My doctor told me that it may take some time before my blood counts normalize. All these chemo treatments (twenty-four in the consolidation phase alone) took a toll on my body. My appointments will start spacing out once my body starts to produce blood on its own. I am so used to having the medical care team monitor me closely, but the responsibility will soon be mine. It's a bit scary to think that, eventually, I will not have the same support I've grown accustomed to this entire time.

On the other hand, it's such a great feeling to know that I'm doing well enough not to need daily, structured assistance. I want to keep my mind in a positive state and might have to remind myself from time to time that I know my body better than anyone. If I ever feel there is a need to contact my doctor before a scheduled appointment due to a concern, so be it.

However, I'll be going back for lab work and seeing my doctor relatively often over the next few weeks. As I heal, we will continue to talk about our plan for the months to come. My faith is overflowing, and I know it will remain strong during this downhill stretch. Hallelujah! Life is almost back to normal! I am at peace.

 Colossians 3:12 ~ Therefore, as God's chosen people, holy and dearly loved, clothe yourselves with compassion, kindness, humility, gentleness, and patience.

THREE

KEEP ON PEDALING

What is life without challenges? If we give up whenever things get complicated, we'll never taste the sweetness of accomplishment. Hold your faith close and let God steer you in the proper direction; as long as you keep pedaling, He will lead you to where you are meant to go.

BLANK SPACES

Your mind will answer most questions
if you learn to relax and wait for the answer.

~ William S. Burroughs

It's January 23, 2015. This week has been full of many trips to the clinic for lab work and blood transfusions. Since receiving my final round of chemo on January 9, I have been experiencing pain on my lower right side, spreading all the way to my back. This lingering pain had not ceased, so I decided to call my doctor. I couldn't tell if the pain was coming from my kidneys, a different organ, or if it was due to something else. I also had some pain around my collar bone on the right side – the same side as my PICC line, and I didn't think that was a good sign either. Perhaps there was a blood clot or something worse? Of course, my mind was rapidly running in circles with dreadful thoughts and worry, even though I had been working on mindfulness and calming strategies. After a couple of phone calls back and forth, my doctor ordered a computed tomography (CT) scan.

My appointment for the CT scan was scheduled for January 21. They took images from my pelvis to my shoulders. This non-invasive procedure took about five minutes from start to finish. I went over to Methodist Estabrook Cancer Center for labs after my CT scan. They ran several tests to check my complete blood count, enzymes, and organ function. I was happy to hear that I did not need a transfusion (yet) and that my enzymes, kidneys, and liver counts looked good. My CT scan results were back as well, and my doctor said that all of my organs looked great. In fact, they couldn't find anything suspicious that would be causing pain. He thought it might be due to tissue or muscle strain. Sometimes not knowing why something uncomfortable is happening is more bothersome than discovering the actual reason. For now, I will continue to have labs two to three times a week until I hear otherwise.

 Exodus 14:14 ~ The LORD will fight for you; you need only to be still.

SPRING INTO ACTION

The food you eat can either be the safest & most powerful form
of medicine or the slowest form of poison.

~ Ann Wigmore

So many unsettling thoughts have been circling in my mind lately. Perhaps it's because my CT scan results left a blank space of more unknowns. I mean, how could there be no rhyme or reason for the cause of my back pain? Now that I think about it, maybe this uncomfortable feeling was triggered by unresolved emotions, most likely because I hadn't dealt with some of the strong feelings associated with my CANcer diagnosis. As I continue to ponder over this thought, I guess there wasn't much time for me to respond upon hearing this news in the first place. Everything happened so fast after confirming that I had acute myeloid leukemia. Naturally, there was an urgency to begin chemo treatments right away since this type of leukemia is very aggressive. Because of that, I had to blindly trust that the medical care team knew how to save my life. I believe a part of me internalized my fears to maintain a more healthy mental balance. It was imperative to continue moving forward in the right frame of mind to boost my chance of survival, even with this fierce awakening of horror and disbelief. Pema Chodron says, "Nothing ever goes away until it has taught us what we need to know." It may be that this unknown cause of pain is trying to get my attention for a specific reason.

Before this diagnosis, I believed that I was a healthy person who made an effort to take care of my body. I did my best to eat right, take vitamins, and exercise regularly. I would have never imagined reaching the point of developing this dreadful disease. Surely not me! From my understanding, anyone can get cancer, and it's just the luck of the draw if chemical changes in your body allow these toxic cells to grow. Triggers can come from the type of environment you're in, what you eat, family history, and other unknown stressors. Cancer develops when cells are damaged and rapidly reproduced. Tumors form because your immune system is unable to identify these cells as harmful, allowing them to mutate and continue multiplying out of control.

Sadly, doctors and researchers are not sure what causes leukemia, so I try to be as proactive as possible on what I CAN do. I took some time to reflect on my situation over the past few months and concluded that I have to stop beating myself up. After all, I came through this like a champion! I also researched how I could improve food choices for my family. We are slowly adjusting what we put in our cupboards and refrigerator. For instance, we eat a lot of fruit, but I never purchased organic before because of its price, and to be honest, I really didn't think it was that big of a deal. I was wrong, and now I buy organic when I can. However, if organic prices are too high, any kind of fruit or vegetable is better than none at all. While searching online, I found both a list of foods to avoid and a selection of cancer-fighting foods to consider adding to our daily meals. These polar opposites are known as 'the dirty dozen' and 'the clean fifteen.' My entire family will benefit from the new food choices in our home! This transition gives me a sense of control over my long-term health.

Now that I've sprung into action by making better health choices, I am already feeling more at ease. Retaking charge of my life helps me recognize that providing a solid foundation of nutrition is the first step in cleansing my mind, body, and soul. Here's to a lifetime of wellness!

 1 Corinthians 10:31 ~ So whether you eat or drink or whatever you do, do it all for the glory of God.

NAVIGATING THROUGH UNCHARTED WATERS

Find ecstasy in life; the mere sense of living is joy enough.

~ Emily Dickinson

Monday, January 25, was an exciting day for me because we noticed that my platelets were rising on their own. As the week progressed, they continued to increase but were still below the normal range. My hemoglobin and white counts remained about the same. That's okay, I'll take any good news that comes my way! So, what does all of this mean? There were no transfusions, and the nurse took my PICC line out on Thursday! She put a bandage on my arm to cover the spot where my PICC line had been and said to keep it on for seventy-two hours (which would have been Sunday). I woke up on Friday morning and noticed the skin around my bandage was blistering, red, and very sore. The same thing happened to my skin when they put in my PICC line in August. We discovered that I was allergic to the first bandage protecting my PICC line. Since I knew that my skin was reacting to this small patch, I removed it and placed a band-aid on the area instead. I am thankful, though, that the PICC line is out. As I navigate all of these ups and downs of the CANcer process, I'm reminded every day that EVERY step, no matter how big or small, is miraculous!

On February 4, I was able to see my doctor. We discussed many things, like taking a high-quality vitamin now that chemo is complete, as well as some of the restrictions I still need to keep in place: I can't go in a pool, hot tub, river, or ocean until further notice. I need to wait to get my yearly physical, and the list goes on. We discussed when I would be able to return to work, and he said it could take anywhere from three to six months for my bone marrow to fully recover from the effects of chemotherapy. My return date will depend on how quickly my body is able to gain back strength. Right now, I'm nearly a month out from my final treatment. He said not to rush into anything and give my body time to heal. On the flip side, he also told me that I am doing remarkably well, and he is very pleased with my results.

We both sense that my leukemia will not return. Throughout my journey, I genuinely feel that miracles have followed me and walked alongside me every step of the way. God gave me the strength to make it through. Initially, I told my family, parents, and brother that I would fight this with all the firepower within and come out on top (with God's help, of course). And now the time has finally arrived – victory is mine! Hallelujah!

CANcer does not define me and will not be the death of me. I keep telling myself to navigate forward with positivity because that's half the battle in this war.

 Psalms 28:7 ~ The LORD is my strength and my shield; my heart trusts in him, and he helps me. My heart leaps for joy, and with my song I praise him.

EYEBROWS AND EYELASHES: GATEWAY TO OUR EMOTIONS?

The greater the crisis, it seems, the swifter the evolution.

~ Elizabeth Gilbert

It's February 8, and just when I thought my hair would continue growing back, I glanced in the mirror and noticed that my eyebrows and eyelashes were almost gone! I rubbed my eyes and took a second look while pinching myself just to make sure I wasn't dreaming, and the moment of truth stared back at me... My eyebrows and eyelashes were vanishing right before my eyes! Too bad it's not the unwanted mustache or chin hair women tend to grumble about. I wanted to retaliate and glue some of my dog's hair on the bald spots but knew that would look even worse. So, I decided to embrace it. After all, I'm healthy! That's the important thing. What's wrong with a few missing lashes and brows anyway?

As I stared in the mirror, examining my lack of hair, I recalled a news segment regarding eyebrows that I had seen several months ago. I always thought that the most recognizable feature on a person was their eyes, but this report says that's not the case. They showed photos of many famous faces without their eyebrows. And again, only this time, the same images without their eyes. Interestingly enough, people are more easily recognized by their eyebrows than their eyes! Another interesting fact: Greeks and Romans favored the unibrow look. If women were born without one, they would apply animal fur above their eyes. I guess gluing my dog's fur onto my eyebrows isn't so far-fetched after all!

Think about it, eyebrows frame the face and broadcast our sincerest feelings. They effortlessly convey when we are excited, angry, surprised, sad, and so forth. If brows are not trimmed properly, adequately shaped, or prominently featured (nonexistent or very light), it can change your facial expression completely. So, whether you prefer thick or thin, arched or full, round or square, or even connected, it's clear that eyebrows tell the world who we are. Where does this leave me now? Fortunately, my eyebrows and eyelashes will grow back soon enough, but until then, does this mean that my emotions and feelings will broadcast differently? Perhaps they will present themselves the same.

Even though my eyebrows were nearly bare for a brief period, I still sense that my family understood my feelings from the tone of my voice. Since I wear my emotions on my sleeve, I am very theatrical when using my words – high or low pitched, monotone, excited, happy, angry, or even sad. My family never said much about it except, "It looks like your eyebrows are getting thicker." Or I would say, "Look, I am wearing mascara again!" And they would chuckle because I only had a couple of strands of lashes to cover. Regardless, it made me feel pretty to apply even one strand with mascara. And that was enough to make me happy.

The week before my initial diagnosis, I remember Colby (fourth grade) and Shaylee (first grade) playing in the basement. I could hear giggles from afar, so I didn't feel the need to check on them. A short while later, Shaylee came upstairs – very upset. It didn't take much time for me to notice that one of her eyebrows was nearly gone! I asked what on Earth happened? She proceeded to tell me that Colby tricked her.

Colby had asked Shaylee if she wanted to shave her eyebrows with him while handing her a razor. He had a fake razor that the boys used when pretending to shave with Tim. Shaylee had a real one and didn't realize it because Colby was showing her (with his fake razor) that it was all just pretend. Needless to say, she actually shaved off her eyebrow. I was so upset with Colby. The school year was going to start in a couple of days. How could he do such a thing? Shaylee was mortified and didn't want to go to school until the hair on her brow grew back. I immediately went to the store and bought an eyebrow pencil that matched her brow color. For two days, I practiced applying the liner to perfect the look by the time she had to go to school.

When school began, Shaylee was very self-conscious about the shave-job and covered that eye with her long hair, even with the eyebrow penciled in. The teacher would tell Shaylee that she couldn't see her eyes, but that didn't stop her from covering it up. A couple of days after school began, I was admitted into the hospital and would remain there for nearly one month. Shaylee was so upset because she didn't think Tim could pencil in her eyebrow, but there was no other option, so she needed to deal with it.

I felt so sorry for her and hoped Colby learned his lesson. Mean or cruel tricks may seem funny to the person behind them, but they can be very hurtful and embarrassing for the victim. I asked Colby to put himself in Shaylee's shoes. How would he like it if this happened to him and HE had to go to school with a fake eyebrow? Shaylee (at her young age) thought they were just pretending, and Colby took his prank too far! It was so disappointing and happened at the worst time – when I couldn't be there to help Shaylee get through it. I was so glad that Holly stepped up and helped cover the bald area with eyeliner when needed. It was a family effort to get Shaylee through this embarrassing episode. And it didn't take long for Colby to realize what he had done, and he felt terrible for tricking her.

Every day (until the brow grew back), Tim diligently drew on an eyebrow for Shaylee to create the illusion of hair. Holly touched it up even more when Shaylee felt like his work wasn't good enough. None of Shaylee's classmates said anything to her, but surely they noticed, especially since Shaylee made a point to cover that eye with her hair for many weeks. Or perhaps Shaylee's inner beauty came out so strong that no one even detected the missing hair. I'd like to believe that's the case. As an adult going through a relatable situation, I had the option of staying home, but Shaylee didn't. She had to face everyone in first grade, fearful of classmates teasing her. I am very proud of Shaylee for continuing to move forward, even when it wasn't easy. A lesson was learned here: Do not believe everything someone says to you, and trust only half of what you see!

Now, our family can laugh about this incident, even Shaylee. She told us there was a reason for covering that eye with her hair. During gym class or outdoor recess, her sweat would cause the liner to run or smear. Shaylee said it was so embarrassing, and she didn't know how to fix it, so she covered it up! I wish Shaylee would have told us. Tim would have gone to the store to find a smudge-free option. I have never been particularly familiar with all the latest makeup trends, tricks, or tips. Who knew there was an option for waterproof brow liner? It was definitely a learning experience for everyone.

Beauty radiates from the inside out, and God created us in His personalized, distinctive fashion. We need to remind ourselves of this artistry as we face daily struggles and challenges. Sometimes we find ourselves putting in a great deal of effort to fit in. So what do I tell myself now? "Relax, Mary. You don't have to try so hard." We are all created perfectly in

God's eyes. Let His light shine through you. Perhaps it will be contagious, just like a smile.

 2 Corinthians 4:17-18 ~ For our light and momentary troubles are achieving for us an eternal glory that far outweighs them all. So we fix our eyes not on what is seen, but on what is unseen, since what is seen is temporary, but what is unseen is eternal.

IF I ONLY HAD A BRAIN

Peace is the result of retraining your mind to process life as it is, rather than as you think it should be.

~ Dr. Wayne Dyer

Most have seen the classic movie *Wizard of Oz* and remember Scarecrow does not have a brain but very much yearns for one. Throughout the movie, Scarecrow displays his ignorance in a fun way but also demonstrates that he already has the brain he so desperately desires. Towards the end of the film, the Wizard recognizes Scarecrow as the wisest man in all of Oz! Scarecrow is so proud and finally realizes that he *does* have a brain, *is* smart, and *has* worth!

I think all of us can relate to Scarecrow and his feelings of not being good enough, thanks to his perceived lack of brains. I know I've done things at one time or another that have made me red-faced from embarrassment. A specific example would be my confused laughter in a group when I don't understand what is so funny. We all feel lost in our own lives sometimes. These feelings can manifest from something as simple as trying to find misplaced keys to something as complicated as an anxiety attack in a public area. The most common experience of mine is walking into a room with a simple task in mind, only to lose track of what I was set out to do. We all experience some type of memory lapse in our lives. And who can blame us with all the pressures of society weighing us down? Struggling to fit in cultivates anxiety and tension that only exacerbates the effects of everyday forgetfulness. When we are under a perceived threat, it is challenging to make even simple decisions.

These everyday hindrances are taken to an entirely new level after going through chemotherapy. Chemo brain, or fog, is one of the top concerns of cancer patients worldwide. It heightens the everyday experience of forgetfulness and can be very counteractive as you are recovering. This fog, or cognitive change, is experienced by most cancer patients who have received chemotherapy or radiation. Simply put, there are times when a person has unexpected difficulties with word recall, short-term memory, concentration, or focus. What does this mean for everyday life? You need to create new pathways in your brain to retrieve memories that would have been easily accessible in the past.

Fortunately, I have not experienced 'heavy-duty' brain fog, like some. Yes, there are moments of pause when I struggle to sort through the piles of words in my head, but my cognition is improving every day. This weight on my brain was most recognizable during and directly after chemo treatments. To normalize my thinking as soon as possible, I proactively enrolled in an eight-week class called *Brain Fog* after my treatments were completed. This class provided valuable strategies to help alleviate the restricting neural symptoms more rapidly. Additionally, participants acquired general information relating to the complexities of our brain's operations. The class was both fascinating and incredibly empowering!

Call to Mind

I am definitely going to take a course on time management...
just as soon as I can work it into my schedule.

~ Louis E. Boone

Over the years, I have personalized many strategies and found that my cell phone calendar is the best tool to help remind me of commitments, keep organized, and stay efficient. Suppose I begin to feel overwhelmed from having too many tasks on any given day. In that case, I take a few deep breaths and prioritize my obligations by importance to reduce my level of anxiety. Occasionally, I take it a step further and break down each task to make them more manageable. Just by doing this, I discovered that I was my worst enemy because I didn't say 'no' to requests when my plate was already full. It occurred to me that I had some control over my schedule, so it was worth my time to simplify it.

In addition to the *Brain Fog* class, Tim and I are involved in a twelve-week program called *A Time to Heal.* This program is for cancer patients who have completed treatments and their caregivers. It's designed to provide support while recovering from cancer and offers encouragement for the person caring for you. We have only met three times so far, but I have thoroughly enjoyed every minute.

One concept gained from *A Time to Heal* is that we all hold some form of resiliency (the ability to bounce back from and successfully overcome risks and adversity). Everyone needs resilience to evolve, and we all have the capabilities to develop flexibility. During class, we wrote down our weaknesses on the left side of a sheet of paper – these are problem areas or anything that holds us back from resolving an issue. Then we wrote our strengths on the right side. This activity is beneficial for anyone wanting to unveil their qualities. Some may need help identifying their strengths (I did) because they have never taken the time to reveal them. Others may not know their strengths at all, and that's okay. If you have difficulty realizing them, a helpful way to look at positive attributes is to ask yourself how a close friend would describe your qualities or even how your pet would describe you (if they could talk). If you still have trouble, do this with a close, trusted friend or family member. They may find this tool valuable for themselves too. And don't underestimate yourself! It seems like people, more often than not, underrate themselves (especially women) rather than overestimating.

Trust me, setting aside a bit of time to make this list of self-discovery has the potential to awaken the best in you. You may even begin to manifest your desires because of this reflection or be inspired to travel into new territory. You might even want to dissolve old thought patterns or weaknesses that have been an unknown hindrance in your successes.

It is only when you begin to utilize your unique strengths that you can reach your fullest potential. Take Scarecrow, for instance, he didn't recognize his value until he was forced to do so and could reflect upon it. Don't we all have a little bit of Scarecrow in us? Our positive assets can be put to good use if we wake up and apply them. So, stand by your individuality! Everything you need is already within.

 Philippians 4:19-20 ~ And my God will meet all your needs according to the riches of his glory in Christ Jesus. To our God and Father be glory for ever and ever. Amen.

REVIVAL SEASON

Nature gives to every time and season some beauties of its own;
and from morning to night, as from the cradle to the grave,
it is but a succession of changes so gentle and easy
that we can scarcely mark their progress.

~ Charles Dickens

Spring is the season of new beginnings, the rebirth of dormant beauty. Time with my family has continued to rejuvenate me. Additionally, absorbing the restorative rays of the sun has boosted my energy. The bright hues of color and mild warmth send positive endorphins throughout my body, mind, and spirit.

The weather is proving itself to be better every day this time of year. Outdoor activities are becoming a daily event at my house. The trees are budding. Birds are caroling sweet melodies in the distance, and every so often, I catch a glimpse of their sleek feathers as they glide gracefully overhead. I revel in this time of year. Something about all the sounds, sights, and warm impressions of spring electrifies my spirit, like when a spark plug ignites an engine. It leaves a lasting impression on my heart, making the day that much brighter.

On March 11, Colby asked me to play soccer. I took advantage of the opportunity to spend quality time with him, and we had fun kicking the ball back and forth. There were lots of laughs and ball chasing! The ball just never seemed to go where we thought it would end up! Then Shaylee asked if we would play basketball with her. We played a game of 'P-I-G' (for Shaylee, it was P-I-G-G-I-E-S, just to give her more chances to score before she lost the game). For anyone who doesn't know the PIG game, it's like HORSE, except a shorter version for those of us who may not want to play the game for as long. The idea of this game involves 'matching' baskets. Each time a player makes a shot, the others need to recreate it from the same position. If they end up missing the shot, a letter is added to their score: beginning with P, then I, and G (in Shaylee's case, P, I, G, G, I, E, S, because she doesn't make the shots too often). The first player who spells PIG is out of the game, and the last person standing wins. We had a good time. It was nice to feel like a kid again.

I have another doctor's appointment on March 18, and I'm actually excited about it! My blood work and stamina have been steadily improving. I'm sure that trend will continue. There is not a day that goes by when I don't stop and pause to thank God for healing me. All the pain and suffering that went along with treating my CANcer is slowly fading into a distant memory. We are fortunate that our brains allow challenging and frightening circumstances to cloud over with time. Hmm… maybe some of the brain fog caused by chemo isn't so bad after all!

Now that I'm feeling healthier, I am blessed to attend church services again. As Matthew West stated, "Christian life was never meant to be lived alone. Together we're a body. A family. The people of God." Amen to that! It has been so enjoyable to see familiar faces and feel their love. In fact, I sat down one day and wrote a short poem about it:

CHURCH

A church is more than just a place of worship.

A church is more than people sitting in pews listening to the Word of God.

A church is a community of Christians who do all they can for someone in need.

A church is unconditional love.

I wrote this simplistic poem from a heart of gratitude. There are no words for the members of our church who have come together to pray on my behalf. It's refreshing to see caring groups of individuals join forces in times of need. The refreshment of a church community is similar to the pleasant feeling of spring's arrival. Just as a strong group of Christians gathers in prayer, divine intervention takes over and blooms a colorful beauty of its own. Foliage and other plant life have processes of growing until maturation. Trees sprout new buds while progressively expanding into leaves, flowers, or fruit. Green stems peek out of the soil and continue to evolve into plentiful harvests. Both prayer and the spring season bring about new growth. Without this unity, I'm not sure that I would be here to expand on my story. We need each other to grow, flourish, and sometimes, as in my case, to live.

Upon further reflection, it occurred to me that each of the four seasons has individual characteristics and revitalizes my soul in its own way. Sometimes a brief dormancy stage, such as winter, is necessary for us to collect ourselves and refocus our goals. This stillness may seem diminutive on the outside, but, in actuality, significant shifts are happening within. The GO, GO, GO mentality of summer is fun, but it's crucial to take timeouts for self-care. We will always be able to circle back after periods of rest. Embrace the transition!

 2 Corinthians 5:17 ~ Therefore, if anyone is in Christ, the new creation has come: The old has gone, the new is here!

ATTITUDE IS EVERYTHING

*Virtually nothing on Earth can stop a person with
a positive attitude who has his goal clearly in sight.*

~ Denis Waitley

We all want to have some control over our lives. Think about it. We can control what we put in our mouths to eat and drink. We can control our way of thinking by choosing to be positive or negative. And thank goodness we have a choice on how we respond to situations and the people involved. We hold the power of all of these things!

On the other hand, there is a lot that we cannot control. Wednesday, March 18, began like any typical day when I headed to Omaha for labs and a doctor's visit. I have not found myself overly anxious or nervous about labs in the past. In fact, I look forward to seeing the staff members who took such good care of me during the past eight months and appreciate seeing that my blood work continues to improve. I find myself tired occasionally, but overall, I feel good. In my mind, these are strong indications of a smooth recovery.

I was welcomed as usual when I arrived at Methodist Estabrook Cancer Center. After labs, I went to my doctor's office and found out that my doctor was out of town, but the nurse practitioner would see me instead. I had only met her once but was okay with it because I felt like everything would be all right anyway.

When she came into the waiting room, we discussed how things had been going and looked over my lab results. My white count and hemoglobin continued to rise, but my platelets were slowly dropping with each visit. A few weeks ago, my platelets were 210,000, then 156,000, and yesterday it was 120,000 (normal range is 150,000-400,000 mcL). I know that I shouldn't let fear control my life, but I have to admit, at that moment – when the nurse practitioner was going over my numbers and expressed that my platelets were still dropping – I became a little nervous, anxious, and let's just say, worried. She also wanted me back in two weeks for labs and another doctor visit just to be on the safe side. She said to do my best not to worry about this because it is normal for white cells, hemoglobin, and platelets to jump around for several months after chemo treatments. However, I continued to let fear and doubt set in my mind. I told her that leukemia had packed its bags and left, and I wanted to keep it that way. In that moment, though, my mind replayed some negative experiences I had from the effects of chemo. I couldn't hold in the big alligator tears any longer. She gave me a tissue, and I began asking several questions. Some of them were: "Is it possible to get another form of leukemia since my other counts are high?" No, she hasn't seen that happen. "Is there anything I can do to help raise my platelet counts?" No. "Would a platelet transfusion 'jumpstart' my body to produce more?" No. I will only get a platelet transfusion if my numbers are too low.

Here was my chance to choose my attitude in a situation where I didn't have control. I decided to rely on faith and the knowledge that this shall pass. However, a good cry is also very cleansing for the soul. Sobbing doesn't mean that I don't have a positive attitude. I'm giving myself compassion on the hard days as I continue to gain strength. My visit didn't go the way I thought it would. I was already celebrating the prediction of hearing good news before my appointment even began! On the drive home, I did my best to set worry aside. I need to keep reminding myself that God has this, and I will rest on His shoulders whenever I need comfort. Yes, it's a fact that my platelets have been decreasing over the past few weeks, but that doesn't mean there's an underlying problem causing it. My blood levels will continue to have a yo-yo effect until they stabilize. I need to remain calm and choose not to surrender my power to fear and doubt.

There are situations in life that I cannot control, such as this one. Thankfully, I *can* control my attitude regarding the power of faith. Perspective is my strength. Some days are more challenging to maintain a hopeful, optimistic attitude than others. Even with my bright outlook, the 'what if' fear always manages to creep into the back of my mind. After all, it's human nature. And just because I'm doing my best to stay positive, no self-assurance is capable of masking the pain that I've experienced. People often deny real emotions with a so-called 'optimistic' attitude, and this avoidance strategy only cultivates more delusion. To continue my faith-filled walk, I'm allowing myself to embrace challenges as life lessons. FAITH and HOPE give me the strength to carry on amidst the pain. The meaning behind those two words is the driving force of my survival.

These days, I remind myself to live in the present and take one day at a time. I try not to worry about what the future holds – I know this is easier said than done. Occasionally, I catch myself in a snag and need to untangle it. Regardless, I am slowly learning that no matter how hard anyone tries, we really don't have control over our future.

I have spent much of my life worrying needlessly over situations I have no control over that end up working themselves out. Sometimes it takes a little more patience, but I know God is in control and working tirelessly for our benefit. I also recognize that staying positive provides comfort in my human body. I have an inner sense of knowing that I CAN-cer-vive! I choose life!

2 Timothy 1:7 ~ For God gave us a spirit not of fear but of power and love and self-control.

STANDING STURDY IN THE STORM

The greater your storm, the brighter your rainbow.

~ Unknown

While driving to an appointment to see my doctor on April 1, I found the tension of my anxiety rising. I searched through radio stations, attempting to find a song that I knew... something that would ease my nerves and spread peace over me. I didn't have much luck, so I let my mind wander. I recalled driving my kids to school recently and asking each one of them how my illness affected them. Holly quickly responded and said that she knew it had to be hard for me to leave our home and be in the hospital for such a long time, so she decided to give up an item that she dearly loved to show her support. Holly said it wasn't fair that I needed to leave our home, so she let go of her favorite blanket that she had slept with since infancy. I never knew Holly did that before our conversation. Her thoughtfulness melted my heart. Brody said that he tried to be a big help for dad when I was away and did what he could to lend a hand around the house. Colby told me that he was sad I got sick and had to go away, but he knew I had to leave if I wanted to stay alive. Shaylee said that she missed cuddles and hugs from me. She also mentioned that it was hard to be happy all the time because she was sad for me.

I reassured my children that no matter what the future held, I would always be a part of them, even in spirit. Life must go on even when the most difficult circumstances happen, and they must have the strength to move forward with a positive outlook. I believe it's critical to discuss feelings with your children when things like this happen, or any time for that matter, so they learn new strategies and gain coping skills to take with them throughout life.

When I arrived at Estabrook, I took advantage of the short walk to the building, assuring myself that everything would be just fine. The sun's warmth reminded me of how good it felt to watch the kids playing in nature the day before. In my mind, I painted a picture of them glancing at me and taking a pause to shout, "Hi, mom!" with a wave of their hand. My kids have a way of calming my nerves like nothing else can. Images of them laughing and enjoying adventures together help me reach a safe haven in my mind. These snapshots give me the strength to move forward in the minefield that stands between me and my health.

There I was, standing at the main door of Estabrook, and told myself to open it. I entered the building and checked in for labs. When the phlebotomist called my name, we walked to a small room. As she inserted the needle into my vein, I noticed a pool of blood began to surround the needle. There was an eerie silence. Such extreme blood loss from a needle-poke had never happened to me before. When my platelets were low in previous circumstances, I had a PICC line for blood withdrawals. The phlebotomist wrapped my arm snuggly when we finished labs, and I walked upstairs to meet with my doctor.

It had been two weeks since my last appointment and the moment of truth that my platelets were decreasing considerably with each visit stared me in the face. That appointment sent my emotions wildly spiraling until they reached the eye of the storm – the zone of calmness. I envisioned my body slowly rotating into the center of the superstorm, and I saw the 'what ifs' trapped in the whirlwind of utter chaos surrounding me. The fierce wind was pulling me in all directions with its uncontrollable power. If I were to lose my balance, it would all come crashing down on me with force and carry me off with the roaring debris trapped in its cyclone. When I managed to take control of this grave imagery, intending to squash the feeling of disarray around me, I looked straight up to heaven and prayed for God to have mercy on me. Then, I recalled the miracle in the hospital. The evening that I had the breath of life and days later learning that I was in remission, just as I had believed. I needed to hold on to that moment and let God's peace wash over me.

My doctor walked into the small room, and I immediately asked him if I should be nervous. He said my platelets dropped again but that it's too premature to be anxious at this point. They had plummeted to 94,000 (normal range 150,000 - 400,000 mcL). He wanted to see me back in two weeks. If my platelets drop again, we will discuss having another bone marrow biopsy. Hearing those words – bone marrow biopsy – sent my heart racing. I tried to hide the fear in my voice and told him, "I don't feel like it's anything to be concerned about. However, I will do whatever's needed IF something is going on," as I snatched a tissue. I couldn't hold in the fearful tears any longer. While sobbing, I told him that I didn't want to even think about going through all the chemo treatments again – everything about it sucked.

I was very distraught and felt comfortable enough to have a total meltdown in front of my doctor. There I was, pouring out all of my anxiety and panic to him – in an attempt to deal with my own feelings of distress before going home to my family. Often, I tell my kids, "I'm fine. Don't worry about me. I'm tough. Let's just get through this." Then ask them questions that lead up to open-ended responses, such as: "How are you doing? How would you describe your feelings about XYZ? Tell me something positive that happened at school today." While behind the scenes, I'm just as frightened as they are at times. It was a moment of truth and release. Maybe even a bit of self-forgiveness too. I couldn't be angry with myself for my situation and would not allow myself to be guilt-stricken any longer from all the unknowns. This illness was not my fault. Before I was born into this world, my path was written in the stars. I had to go through this for my soul to evolve. I understand that now. As tears stopped rolling down my cheeks and I regained my composure, I told my doctor that I wouldn't hesitate to do it all over again if it meant that I would have more time with my family. He gave me a sincere hug before I walked out the door.

Regardless of my emotional state (at any given time), I'm doing the best I can with the cards I've been dealt – right or wrong. What matters most is that my children know the importance of talking about their feelings to avoid a charged explosion because they are not dealing with complex situations that may not be pleasant. Sometimes reports (of any kind) catch us off-guard, and we need to find a way to deal with the unexpected news.

For now, I will wait and continue to pray for the best scenario. Even though I tend to deal with my feelings reasonably well, sometimes I burst into a deep emotion-filled panic. And that's okay. I just keep on pedaling until I reach my final destination, sometimes riding on a tandem bike with God steering.

What are some strategies you use to help you get through challenging situations? Some of my methods to deal with feelings are:

- Prayer requests of any kind
  - ○ sometimes I also ask God for a sign and keep my eyes open to receive it
- Meditation with uplifting music, visualizations, and imagery
- Emotional Freedom Technique (EFT) Tapping to help relieve stress and anxiety
- Journaling: writing my feelings on paper
- Affirmations
- Mindfulness and present-moment practice: appreciation of what is right here in the moment
- Finding humor in everyday occurrences
- Watching an uplifting movie or comedy
- Reading a book, magazine, article, inspirational quotes, or scriptures in the Bible
- Maintaining a positive attitude, even when I need to put an encouraging spin on the situation

 Philippians 4:6-7 ~ Do not be anxious about anything, but in every situation, by prayer and petition, with thanksgiving, present your requests to God. And the peace of God, which transcends all understanding, will guard your hearts and your minds in Christ Jesus.

Desperate Times Call for Desperate Measures

I held onto faith and hope in an attempt to keep worry at bay for the next two weeks. I reminded myself (more than once a day) that I felt really good. My white counts and hemoglobin continue to rise with each blood test. Even so, prayers for more platelets were a must. Perhaps my new norm for platelets will be lower than the normal range? I'd be okay with that as long as my platelets reach a plateau and stop dropping. Regardless, I needed to take action – and fast – to find a way for my platelets to rise before my next appointment. This task seems impossible. But is it *really*? As usual, a little divine intervention led me to the right people.

I've always been a resourceful kind of gal. When troubles are brewing, and nothing I do seems to be working, I look to other resources to find a way to solve the situation or at least calm it in some manner. Of course, first and foremost: I always take problems or worries to God and pray for guidance. I'm sure God is the one who led me to the help I needed.

I have a friend who helps people relieve various conditions through the treatment of neurofeedback. When I was first diagnosed with acute myeloid leukemia, he called me to offer support to help my family (and me) get through this difficult time. Additionally, he asked if he could do brain mapping, or Quantitative Electroencephalography (qEEG), on me after each round of chemotherapy treatments for research purposes. He wanted to see how my brain would react to the chemotherapy drugs. He found that my brain was very inflamed (cranky) before chemo treatments began, but it became less and less inflamed after each week-long round. Such a crazy discovery! My body was taking in poisonous chemo treatments, and, for the most part, my brain was showing progress after each drug administration. The only thing that set my neurofunction back was the chemo brain, or brain fog, that began to appear on the qEEGs. After I completed all my rounds of chemo, we decided to go ahead and treat my brain fog directly (with my doctor's permission). With this treatment plan, my qEEGs continued to show improvements in my cognitive processes.

After the appointment with my doctor on April 1, I stopped by this friend's place to catch up and asked if he could help my platelet count rise. Simply put, he said, "No." However, he got on the Internet and started talking about spleens. We read that spleens can harbor platelets. I perked up and said, "You are a genius! That's it! I have two spleens (which I found out from an ultrasound while in the hospital – the extra spleen is called an accessory spleen). I bet my spleens are harboring my platelets, so I probably have a gazillion of them!" I left my friend's place with a bounce in my step and a song in my heart. I was already on my next mission to figure out what I would do with this encouraging news.

At this time, Tim and I had been to ten sessions of *A Time to Heal* and only had two more left. Thus far, we loved this program and learned a great deal of helpful information. About one and a half months prior, a presenter came to the discussion group (as they often did) and talked about ways to calm yourself or others. She is a professional counselor, nationally certified therapeutic massage, and bodyworker. This presenter had extensive knowledge about healing your inner core and provided information about the healing modality of Reiki – a Japanese technique for stress reduction and relaxation that also promotes healing. I thoroughly enjoyed this particular session and asked for her phone number before leaving. She gladly opened my class reference book and wrote her contact information on a random page. Then she told me to be sure I let her know that I was from *A Time to Heal* class if I was ever to phone her. I thought a lot about contacting her but never made the call.

When I got home, I told Tim what had happened at my friend's place and thought this same presenter could help me with my platelets. He said, "Call her!" So that's what I did, and she agreed to meet with me on April 6, which gave me nine days before my doctor's appointment. When I met with this Reiki Master, I told her about my platelet situation and what my friend found out about platelets and spleens. I also mentioned that I have two spleens. She said that was key and agreed that my spleens were holding my platelets! This Reiki healer told me to literally talk to my spleens (in a relaxing, focused state of mind) and kindly ask them to release platelets. It was crucial for me to visualize my spleens releasing platelets into my bloodstream. I was super excited to hear this and went home with a grateful heart and more hope than ever.

As I was meditating on releasing platelets, I thought of guided imagery. Did you know that our bodies can't tell the difference between what is actually happening to us and what we are vividly imagining? Strange as it sounds, it's true. So, I decided to imagine hot little cowboys lassoing platelets that are in my spleens and tossing them into my bloodstream to raise my platelet count to 228,000 mcL (that's the number I chose). Again, I had nine days before my next appointment. Unfortunately, I ended up being very sick with a stomach bug for five of the days, so I had very little nutritional value going into my system during that time. But, guess what? My platelets went from 94,000 to 105,000 at my appointment on April 15! Yes, a rise of eleven points (remember, my platelets had decreased twenty to thirty points with each appointment over the last couple of months). God is so good for nudging me to connect with other resources to help overcome challenges. As I said before, God answers prayers in mysterious ways. Nothing is impossible with Him. Ride 'em, cowboy!

On April 29, I was thrilled with my lab results. Since my last visit, my platelets went up another twenty-six points (131,000 platelets)! Now I was almost within the normal range, only nineteen more points to get there! There was no questioning that the cowboys were efficiently doing their job. It was definitely a day of celebration for us! You better believe that I am still praying to God AND talking to my spleens – yes, BOTH spleens. I wouldn't want to make one of them jealous! Haha... Yee-haw, ride on cowboys!

 Romans 12:2 ~ Do not conform to the pattern of this world, but be transformed by the renewing of your mind. Then you will be able to test and approve what God's will is — his good, pleasing and perfect will.

PAVING THE WAY TO A FULFILLED LIFE

There'll be two dates on your tombstone and all your friends
will read 'em but all that's gonna matter
is that little dash between 'em.

~ Kevin Welch

We all deserve to be happy. It's now the end of April, and I've been thinking about what makes a person happy. What is it that ignites the fire inside someone with such force that it invigorates the soul, leaving them fulfilled, refreshed, and recharged? I have been doing some soul-searching to discover what activates my inner spark and intensifies my upbeat attitude. Why not find what makes each of us happier today? As Louis E. Boone expresses so frankly, "The saddest summary of a life contains three descriptions: could have, might have, and should have." Regrettably, I feel like some of my life experiences have agreed with this reference.

Appearances expertly reflect wealth, beauty, and power, but they have no influence on our internal framework. Sadness, guilt, and shame are just a few emotions that can be stored deep within, never peeking outside the walls built around them. I began to wonder why I'm so scared to move forward with some adventures or remain tight-lipped when I have something important to say on a particular subject? Why am I constantly worried about what others may think of me? Why haven't I outgrown this superficial behavior yet?

The answer is simple in my case. When I was an adolescent, I had an experience with peers that negatively influenced my life. This bullying wounded my character, and it all went downhill after that. It was a case of popularity and jealousy that commonly infiltrates middle and high school friendships. Following that corrosive time in my life, I still have trouble with stressing about fitting in and exuding people-pleasing tendencies. It seems like when I have opportunities to expand relationships into a deeper connection, a part of me shies away from the uncertainty that's to come. This avoidance makes me question if loneliness makes me happier.

My reclusive behavior seems to have started after I moved from my hometown and had a family of my own. It became difficult for me to grow close to people, as being vulnerable often leaves me with hurt feelings. I vowed that my wall would never come down again. Over the years, however, I've had some self-reflection. It seems like this facade is not only blockading my relationships, but also compromising my integrity. I have many gifts to offer and shouldn't hold myself back for fear of being chastised for my way of thinking. It's a lonely world when perfectionism and anxiety block the development of friendships. God created all life in the likeness of Him. Every person on Earth has a purpose and is loved equally. This game of pretend ends now.

With that in mind, I often wonder if I can make my way back to the carefree child I once was. This reminiscing reminds me of the time I received the first level of Reiki with the same Reiki Master/Teacher introduced to us at the *A Time To Heal* session. During the attunement ceremony back in May, I had the most breathtaking vision. I was frolicking happily in a field of tall grass and wildflowers with my arms widely spread and raised toward heaven. I saw myself smile and laugh with immense joy, spinning slowly with each step. There was a gentle breeze, and I felt the warm rays of sun on my face as I soaked in all the light and love. Tears welled up and overflowed, streaming down my cheeks and cleansing my inner soul. After the vision ceased and the ceremony ended, I told the Reiki Master/Teacher of my revitalizing experience. She said I had glimpsed my core being and now understand my true essence. I couldn't believe how beautiful I am inside. Spiritual goosebumps crawled up my arms with this affirmation of truth. That moment marked the beginning of my transformation. Holding onto the memory of me being so joyful and carefree gave me the courage to step forward with a new perspective in my faithful journey. I AM worthy of all desires and have a passion for life.

It takes a while to find the new normal after CANcer. I'm not the same person I was before and have changed for the better in many ways. Life alterations can change a person's perspective in a blink of an eye and move them in a different direction, possibly toward a new goal or adventure. I learned that normal is what you make of it. I am the one who possesses the power and freedom of choice. I will not sit around waiting for happiness to stumble across my path years down the road. I want enjoyment now.

Honestly, some things that made me happy before this battle with CANcer do not interest me now, and life is too short not to make a change. Of course, I'm not telling you to quit your job to rediscover yourself. There is a way to find time for simple pleasures within the busy schedules of today's society.

As I learned from *A Time to Heal* class, you can take steps to create a more fulfilling life. First, define what happiness means to you before looking for it. Sometimes our culture has a very narrow view of happiness, restricting it to superficial possessions. Broadening your perspective helps you understand where you are going and provides a clearer image of your goals.

To me, true joy involves contentment, freedom, overcoming challenges with proficiency, and putting forth great effort. These components of joy can take several different forms in our lives. Sometimes happiness is having the luxury to do nothing for a block of time. Other times, happiness looks like doing something you're passionate about, learning something new, or even volunteering to help others. We are most happy when we can just *be*. In my case, comfort is maximized by a completely empty schedule. If I could, I would enjoy warm drinks with a soft, cozy blanket and my dog every day of the week. Currently, I am working to balance a life that I love with the not-so-fun responsibilities of work.

Research proves that forming positive social connections and enjoying yourself strengthens the immune system. Lord knows I need that! Dr. Lawrence LeShan wrote the book *Cancer as a Turning Point*. He has an interesting approach to surviving cancer and provides strategies that tell your immune system your life is worth fighting for. Add passion to your life and discover true happiness. For instance, let's say you want to go on a lavish vacation but don't have the money. No need to worry – just visualize happy memories or use your imagination. These reflections are just as health-promoting as taking an actual vacation. Remember, the body doesn't know the difference between real and fantasy. Use this to your advantage!

Here it goes: I'm imagining palm trees swaying with the gentle breeze of eighty-degree weather on a bright sunny day. Seagulls are squawking and soaring above the ocean, scoping out the beaches for abandoned edibles to snack on. I'm lounging on a comfortable chair, shaded by an umbrella on the warm sandy beach. The crashing waves periodically strike the shoreline with force. All is well in my world. Tim and the kids are in the near distance, splashing with laughter in the clear salty water. Oh, a refreshing coconut drink with a straw and decorative cocktail umbrella would be an excellent addition! Now that's what I call: Living the good life!

A snorkeling experience with a vast array of brilliantly colored fish, coral reefs, sea turtles, and stingrays would be a lovely vision too! Just the feeling of floating amongst the most beautiful sea creatures in crystal clear water makes my heart overflow with joy. I've actually been snorkeling a few times because our family enjoys it so much. One snorkeling experience was especially memorable, and I have taken myself back to that moment many times in my mind. I was just past the shoreline, snorkeling in the most exquisite coral reef, surrounded by an array of sea creatures. Without thinking, I noticed myself making humming sounds to affirm my satisfaction and praise for this special moment. The restriction of the snorkel in my mouth did nothing to muffle my excitement. I ever so gently swam forward and continued my exploration. I took a deep breath and dove down into a school of angelfish, with hopes of making a connection in some way, perhaps through touch. As I swam further beneath the shallow waters, the school of angelfish parted ways and allowed me to glide between them. It was as if God's angels were surrounding me with their love. Our eyes instinctively met and held no judgment for each other. There was a trust between the angelfish and me that was unexpected. I was in their territory, and they allowed me to swim alongside them without hesitation.

What does 'living a good life' mean to you? How can you discover what your happiness is? The truth is, I can't tell you. Each of us holds the key to our own door of wellness – we have the power to create the future we wish to see. What are you going to use to unlock *your* door?

 John 8:12 ~ When Jesus spoke again to the people, he said, "I am the light of the world. Whoever follows me will never walk in darkness, but will have the light of life."

FOUR

I AM BLOOMING,
AND I WON'T HIDE
IN THE SHADOWS

I'll never get over the magic of how a tiny seed is able to develop into something so elaborate! It could sprout into a watermelon, a tomato, or even an entire tree. Whatever the result, however, the seedling can only survive and flourish if nurtured in a suitable environment; threatening weeds and pests attempting to steal the plant's nutrients need to be managed.

This idea can be paralleled with the growth of humans as well. We all have a bit of pruning to do in our lives – don't let weeds overpower the good seeds you sow. Surround yourself with people who will nurture you, inspire you to be your best, and keep you moving in the right direction.

THE NATURE OF GRAVITY

Please take responsibility for the energy you bring into this space.

~ Dr. Jill Bolte Taylor

Do you ever wonder how some events in life occur? Or why wild organisms are programmed to do specific tasks? When it comes to the complexity of nature, the life of a bee is a perfect example. On the surface, their agenda is simple. However, their daily practices are focused, intentional, and complex. Bees are essential to humanity as they pollinate flowers, encourage growth, and provide versatile honey. Their productions are multifaceted – yields can heal common ailments and add a yummy taste to foods and drinks. Honey, while easily accessible in our neighborhood convenience store, comes from great demands and hard work within the bees' hives.

Let's picture for a moment that a bee somehow flew its way inside a rocket just before takeoff into outer space. It was secretly in the presence of some of the wisest astronauts and learned very quickly that, without gravity or opposition, it no longer needed its wings to fly. In fact, the bee found itself floating gracefully throughout the spaceship with no effort at all. Since the bee had no need to transport itself, it became lazy, going about each day without a care in the world; it floated around in the spacecraft without a mission of its own. As the days went by, the bee grew weaker and weaker. Eventually, as the bee lacked purpose and motivation, its body failed to support itself, and it died a meaningless death.

The moral of this story is that you need to pursue your prospects with intentional force and refuse to settle when things get easy. Opposition isn't even the greatest challenge – the true obstacle is fear. And if you don't combat that fear, you may find yourself like the bee, just floating in space, ignoring the fact that there is work to be done. Although fear is the most significant restriction, impulsivity hinders growth at nearly the same rate. Jumping onboard without considering the consequences can steer your life in an undesired direction. Flaws and misjudgments are natural, but it is necessary to release them, manifest desires on your journey, and have faith in your abilities.

With this in mind, gravity has the power to work with us and against us simultaneously. Gravitational force can be what keeps us grounded through each restriction. On the other hand, the burdens of conflict, or opposition, can also bring us to our knees. Wouldn't it be nice to go about life just floating around like the bee in space, never having to work for anything? One may think so, but sometimes the struggle makes us stronger. Gravity, and other trials, gives us the ability to fulfill God's purpose. Faith evolves each time we practice it, just as our strength increases with exercise. Effort equates to progress.

I wanted more than anything for my platelets to rise during *my* trials. I prayed for wisdom and visited several other resources to help me find the answers I needed. God guided me in the direction of my goal. At my appointment in May 2015, labs were drawn, and I waited patiently for my doctor to come into the room with the results. I was thrilled when he told me that my platelet count was 158,000 (normal range is 150,000–400,000 mcL), hemoglobin was 14.7 grams per deciliter (normal range for women is 12.0–15.5 gm/dL), and white blood cell count was 4,700 (normal range is 4,500–11,000 mcL). I literally jumped up and down in the room and joyfully thanked God. This small bit of normalcy was so refreshing. My doctor told me that whatever I was doing was working and recommended that I remain active in my intuitive routine. I was doing so well that he scheduled my next appointment for two months from that day instead of the regular two weeks. I will continue to do everything in my power to maximize good health, even if that means talking to my spleens and those hot little cowboys. For me, the message I received here is: Ask for help when you need it, believe that you will receive it, and keep the faith.

 Colossians 3:17 ~ And whatever you do, whether in word or deed, do it all in the name of the Lord Jesus, giving thanks to God the Father through him.

OUT LIVING LIFE

In the end, we only regret the chances we didn't take,
the relationships we were afraid to have,
and the decision we waited too long to make.

~ Lewis Carroll

This summer, I embarked on a surprise adventure. It was one that I had never dreamed of taking the time to do before. The events that led to this unforeseen journey all began on May 2. Tim and I went to the first *Art of Living Beyond Cancer Conference* in Omaha. It is sponsored by *A Time to Heal* (the twelve-week program that Tim and I attended after completing all of my chemo treatments).

The day was filled with laughter, hope, and inspirational stories. They had several booths with fliers, free handouts, and informative brochures promoting various programs. One of the programs that piqued my interest was called *First Descents*, and it just so happened that Tim and I sat across from two individuals involved in that organization during lunch. They began sharing all about their adventures in this program. They recommended applying to go surfing, whitewater kayaking, rock climbing, or ice climbing. *First Descents* is for cancer survivors (and other serious health conditions) between the ages of eighteen and thirty-nine. I should mention that there is also a forty to forty-five age category with the same types of adventures. *First Descents* is stationed out of Colorado but offers nationwide cancer-survivor retreats.

I didn't need to think twice about which activity I wanted to do. Kayaking was my choice above the rest. I love to be around (or in) any body of water. In my younger years, my dad took my brother and me fishing as often as time allowed. Sometimes we would even swim in ponds, lakes, or rivers before going home. We always had a good time, even if we didn't get one bite on our fishing line the entire day. I remember how my dad was always brave and unlodged the line whenever it snagged on a branch or got stuck in deep water. Matt and I would get a good laugh as my dad stripped down to his underwear and marched with confidence into the murky water to untangle the mess we made. Naturally, we also made sure to cheer him on and give accolades when he returned with the hook and bobber.

As I got older, my friends and I would travel an hour to Lake Angostura, South Dakota. We enjoyed sunbathing on the sandy beach and splashing in the lake to cool off. I have always wanted to try kayaking but never had the opportunity. The more I thought about this kayaking adventure, the more excited I became.

For years, I witnessed people leisurely floating down the Platte River in kayaks. They're always happy to shout a greeting to us as the current pushes them along. I would like to think that they see endless bursts of wildlife from their prime position on the rippled water, and I can't wait to take my turn!

I wondered if *First Descents* also offers unique self-soothing strategies to help ease anxiety. I'm very interested in the techniques that calm the spirit. Acting on this thought, I decided that it was time to officially book a trip. Looking deeper into the brochure, it turns out that this popular program has a waiting list. It wasn't too worrisome, however, because I saw that I could still get in THIS season if I took action quickly.

I got home and immediately checked the website. I thought, "Could this really be free? A week-long adventure, staying at a lodge with other cancer survivors, two chefs cooking fresh organic meals, and learning to kayak, surf, or climb! Wow, where do I sign?" I filled out the online application and submitted it. In no time at all, I heard back from a *First Descents* member with news of my acceptance into the program! They told me to take my pick of any dates, locations, or adventures. That is IF my doctor approves of the challenge.

Without hesitation, I called my doctor's nurse and left a detailed message about this trip opportunity, along with my preference to go whitewater kayaking. I included that I would be more than willing to take on the rock climbing adventure if my doctor didn't want me in the river. Since the leukemia diagnosis, I have not been able to go in any pools, hot tubs, rivers, lakes, or other bodies of water that could compromise my immune system. Fortunately, the nurse called me back shortly after I left the message and said my doctor approved the kayaking trip. She jokingly said, "But only if he could go too!" It was such an exciting moment for me. I leaped so high with joy that I almost dropped my phone!

I chose to leave on July 19, a date as close to August as possible, to give my body about two more months to continue healing. I needed to complete a few more steps before the *First Descents* trip could be approved. First, I had to choose the kayaking location and have my doctor complete a physical form. Next, I had to follow up with additional documents and waivers. Finally, when all that messy work was done, I could purchase my plane ticket (I want to mention that there were airfare scholarships for those who needed assistance). I had been wanting something to look forward to ever since this CANcer scare, and now was my big opportunity.

July 19 seemed to come quickly. That day, I flew into Albany, New York and met with two *First Descents* crew members and some other CANcer survivors. I was a bit nervous about meeting new people but did my best to hide the apprehension behind my smile and our introductions. We drove two hours to reach our destination at the lodge in Charlemont, Massachusetts, which provided more time for our small group to connect. The view was breathtaking! I had never seen so many rolling hills with luscious forests and stunning rock formations.

The landscape around the lodge was practically an oasis, provoking tranquil feelings deep within my soul. Colorful prayer flags were hanging from the tree limbs at our retreat lodge. These flags are believed to be activated by the wind. It is common to write a person's name, birth date, or wedding date on prayer flags to personalize it. Prayers, symbols, and mantras can be added to the flags. It is said that blessings are released as the wind carries the prayers from the cloth into the heavens. And with each of these holy transfers, the fabric frays and the printed images on the flags fade. When the flags are well worn, they are often burned to send off the last expression of prayer. It is also common to see old, tattered flags beside new ones, left to the elements.

We parked the van, unloaded our belongings, and met the rest of the group. All ten of us women became close quickly (we were told it was not common to have only females). Each morning began by eating a delicious breakfast and packing a nutritious lunch to enjoy at the river. Then we drove along windy stretches of the pristine terrain to experience a week of kayaking on various points of the Deerfield River. The layers of green woodlands and grasslands were alive with natural beauty. Along the road were brief sightings of the river rapids with large boulders scattered about. We saw several groups paddling their kayaks with the strong current, navigating around jagged rock formations. This intense kayaking looked like great fun, but we weren't headed to that part of the river rapids until later in the week. Our first few days began at nearby calm bodies of water. The instructors thought it was necessary that we train and develop basic skills before launching into the more advanced, potentially dangerous parts of the river. The crew tested our balance in the kayaks with water games. Each day, we learned paddling strategies and progressed to more challenging waters after achieving each milestone. These practices were all leading up to the full escapade in the whitewater rapids.

The next few days gave me more perspectives regarding attitude, courage, and strength. Although I can't speak definitively for all the women who attended this trip, it seemed like some of us came in a weaker state than others. Perhaps we were a little fearful of kayaking, meeting new people, or had recently finished treatments. Regardless, everyone seemed to have left feeling strong and brave for all our hard work throughout the week. It was also apparent that some just came for an adventure, like me! In addition to that, though, I was also hoping this trip would help me move past my lingering anxiety. It never hurts to learn new strategies and expand your resources.

I knew I was strong and brave for having gone through CANcer, but that was for survival and certainly not something I would wish to do again. I wanted to internally prove that I had the courage to step out of my comfort zone independently. That means making decisions for myself, far away from the support of my loved ones. I accomplished my goal with this trip! *First Descents* allowed me to meet new people in a different state far from my support system, speak freely even if I felt vulnerable, and, all-around, try something new. These introductions led to the self-discovery that I CAN do anything if I intentionally set my mind to achieve it.

All the women on this journey had at least one thing in common: We are fighters and SURVIVORS. Each of us understood the feelings that come with a cancer battle. Every evening, we were faced with deep conversations around a bonfire and played games that involved sharing personal information or experiences. Of course, we had the choice of passing to the next person, but all of us were comfortable enough to expose pieces of ourselves. I'd like to think these activities also played a role in our healing process. Not to mention, every woman was awarded a prize by the end of the week for their 'awesomeness!' Each day, the leaders chose two women who overcame a challenge or demonstrated bravery during our kayaking ventures. The winners were handed a plastic shelled bikini top or Hawaiian shorts to wear until they had to transfer the fashionable prizes to the next day's lucky pair of women. It sure felt nice to be recognized for a courageous, independent action taken on the water. These symbolic tropical artifacts were perfect reminders of the bravery each of us women demonstrated throughout the week. For me, it was very uplifting and kept my motivation moving full speed.

Undoubtedly, spending time on the rocky whitewater and successfully maneuvering through hefty currents made me forget about my current weakened state. It was amazing to see our group grow in physical, emotional, mental, and even spiritual strength that week. Yes, there were moments with scary situations, tears, bumps, and bruises, but none of those nuances brought anyone down. With each flick of our paddles, we zoomed past any struggle or trial that came our way. Just as we all had done while fighting CANcer, we refused to let the stream divert us from our line of travel.

The final day of kayaking was our moment of truth. The strong current looked even more frightening close up, but the intensity also made me feel alive. All of us championed through the rapids. At one point, however, my kayak hit a large boulder, and I flipped over! For a few seconds, I was consumed with worry as the frothy rapids engulfed me. Thanks to pure instinct, I somehow managed to flip myself upright again, just as a crew member was coming to my rescue. It was an exhilarating feeling of victory, and everyone in the group gave cheerful support for my success. We were in this together. At that moment, there was nothing that could take our power away, not even the thrashing, whipping, and unforgiving surge of the current. As we made it past the danger zone and reached slower-paced water, I gazed around at our group and wondered if we would maintain our friendships from afar. I contemplated what life would look like for each of us upon returning home. Then I smiled crookedly, held my paddle high in the air, and shouted a loud *ROAR!* This moment was dedicated completely to God. I know what it feels like to overcome fear. This trip left me feeling confident, triumphant, and fulfilled.

 John 10:10 ~ The thief comes only to steal and kill and destroy; I have come that they may have life, and have it to the full.

STRUGGLES BRING TRIUMPHS

*Gratitude unlocks the fullness of life. It turns what we have
into enough, and more. It turns denial into acceptance,
chaos to order, confusion to clarity. It can turn a meal
into a feast, a house into a home, a stranger into a friend.*

~ Melody Beattie

We all know there are bound to be changes in the weather patterns
and natural world with each season – spring, summer, fall, and winter.
Similarly, our lives also go through phases of development throughout our
lifetime – sprouting, blooming, expanding, and simply existing in an idle
state. Everyday challenges arise as we evolve from these changes, whether
we like it or not. There are moments of joy, laughter, tears, and struggles.
All of these moments have the potential to significantly impact our next
steps, along with affecting our intrinsic human nature. Amid challenging
times, we need to remember that struggles make us stronger and wiser in
the end.

We've all gone through periods of hopelessness, confusion, and self-
doubt. Too often, we push away these negative emotions instead of embracing
them. Society is more comfortable with cheerful and positive behaviors, so
it's only natural to conform to suppression. It takes a tremendous amount
of effort and energy to try to be something we're not. Emotions always seem
to find their way out in the end, anyway. And the longer we hold them
in, the more explosive their release seems to be. I believe that *all* feelings
exist to teach us life lessons – to grow us physically, emotionally, mentally,
and spiritually. Our persona revolves around a core of internal truth – the
perceptions of those around us mean nothing.

It's sometimes difficult to hear about the challenges of others because
similar situations can bring up some of *our* unresolved feelings. Additionally,
spouses and friends try to seek solutions for us without understanding the
source of the *real* problem. Maybe it's because they don't want to see the
person they care about in pain. Or perhaps *our* struggles are just more
reminders of the same issues in *their* lives. Everything feels like a projection.

Most of us tend to jump to the rescue in desperate times to relieve anxieties about situations – and sometimes there is a need for that, but are we *really* helping that person in the long run? Or are we just trying to help ourselves? The best thing to do for a friend in need is to listen, advise, and support. We need to be present and grant them full freedom in finding a solution. Sometimes all a person needs is for someone to hear them. Talking through a situation works wonders.

A friend of mine shared a fascinating story with me. She told me that a baby chick in an egg will struggle to get out of the hard shell. The chick uses its beak to peck itself out and must go through this process because it needs to develop strength. The hatchling must peck and toil to get out of the shell, which can take anywhere from hours to days. It takes perseverance and power for a chick to crack through an egg. If a person uses *their* strength to take the chick out of its shell, the chick will surely die. Just like chicks need resistance to become strong, humans need opposition to evolve. So, keep on pecking when struggles seem to take a long time to resolve.

My family and I had a taxing year with my CANcer scare, but I learned to embrace it. CANcer has taught me that I have so much more strength than I ever could have imagined. I have learned incredible lessons about compassion, relying on faith, and perseverance. Why did it take such a difficult circumstance to teach me these lessons? I'll never know the exact reason, but maybe that chick and I have something in common – we both needed to struggle before we could develop strength for life. Perhaps this whole process is like giving birth – you have to go through a lot of pain, but in the end, you have a miracle!

In August 2015, we celebrated the grand opening of the Sensory Courtyard with a Chamber Ribbon-Cutting Ceremony. The turnout was fantastic! It meant so much to see my project in all its glory. I also went to the doctor this same month. My blood work was the best it's been since remission. My doctor and I were ecstatic! He didn't know if my complete blood count would ever be in the normal range again since most aren't after battling CANcer. Fortunately, the results of my blood work have continued to improve.

I don't have to go back for lab work until October. The distance between appointments is lengthening, and it sure feels good. God has healed me and blessed me in this challenging time. I have a new appreciation for the little things life has to offer, like watching my kids' faces light up when they've earned a reward, hearing about their day and what made them smile, or working with my students and seeing their proud expression when they learn something new. Life is good, and God is awesome! Ahh, what a difference a year can make! There is hope, love, and joy weaved into the lining of every seasonal struggle.

 James 1: 2-3 ~ Consider it pure joy, my brothers and sisters, whenever you face trials of many kinds, because you know that the testing of your faith produces perseverance.

SOAKING IN THE BLESSINGS

A woman who walks in PURPOSE
doesn't have to chase people or opportunities.
Her LIGHT causes people and opportunities to pursue HER.

~ Unknown

I've been showered with blessings for the past few months, and it's such a delight to reflect on all the good. I firmly believe that having a positive mindset contributed significantly on the road to my rewarding outcome. When I was in the throes of my CANcer experience, I never would have dreamed of the godsends that were to come. Perhaps my optimistic state of mind brought more than just good health. Maybe my certainty of survival also came from manifesting other favors to come my way. Regardless, there's no reason to search for the truth of life — we can find the answers within ourselves.

Moments of Time

It's already October, and I now see my doctor every three months to get my blood levels checked. This month's checkup went well. My counts were almost the same as last time, but they dropped slightly. My blood work is still within the normal range, and that's all that matters to me at this point. Of course, I was a little concerned that my counts had declined, but my doctor assured me that I was doing fantastic. This blood sample was just a moment in time, and results will always vary, to some extent, with each visit.

Before the checkup with my oncologist, my family had eye exams. In the past, we had been very good about checking our vision on a yearly basis, but last year we dropped the ball. When I saw my eye doctor, she was shocked to hear that I had leukemia the previous year. We discussed that sometimes eye doctors can tell if a patient has cancer just from a routine eye exam. If something out of the ordinary shows up during the slit lamp or retinal examination, they refer patients to their family doctor for blood work. I found this to be a fascinating fact. Signs of ill health can display themselves anywhere on our body – even the eyes.

During my eye exam, the eye doctor told me that I had retinal hemorrhages in the lower-back portion of both eyes. These bursts occur when abnormal bleeding is present in the retina's blood vessels. Retinal hemorrhages have many causes, including diabetes, high blood pressure, anemia, and leukemia. My eye doctor said she wasn't too worried about them since I frequently visit my oncologist. She said my body has been through a lot, and it's not surprising that it reacted. My eyes will be rechecked in a year unless I choose to go to an ophthalmologist for a second opinion. Hopefully the hemorrhaging will resolve itself. I am doing my best to keep moving forward without worry.

I talked to my oncologist about the eye exam findings, and he asked if I had flown on a jet recently… and I had! I flew to Kentucky the week before my eye appointment. My doctor thinks the pressure from the flight may have had something to do with it. We will continue to monitor my blood work closely. If I get too uneasy about it, he said I could always go to an ophthalmologist to confirm my condition. For now, God's presence is the only confirmation I need.

Au Revoir, Friends

It's December 1. Tim and I went to the six-month reunion for the *A Time to Heal* program. This gathering was a final conclusion to the twelve-week sessions we had from February to May in 2015. I was eager to converse with everyone from our group and find out how they've been. Several came to the reunion and had incredible stories to share. Some had returned to work, taken precious time out for hobbies and loved ones, or traveled to exotic places. Others were still struggling with CANcer – either from it returning or spreading. We were also given the terrible news that an admirable woman from our class lost her battle to cancer. Her death was really unsettling to me. This 'reality check' reminded me that my time on earth is precious. No one knows how long they have in this world, so I will do my best to prioritize the time God has granted me.

Patient Perspective

I was thrilled to get an email from a staff member at Methodist Hospital asking me to present to healthcare providers and supporting personnel on January 18, 2016. She wanted me to share my personal experience with the CANcer diagnosis, treatment, and follow-up. The doctors want to familiarize themselves with the patients' perspectives. This same woman gave me information for the *A Time To Heal* twelve-week program (that Tim and I enjoyed so much). She wears many hats in her position and helps coordinate educational experiences for their stem cell transplant organization. This year, the organization's focus was on acute myeloid leukemia, hence why they asked me to present.

Even though I didn't receive a stem cell transplant, she thought I would have a lot to offer to the health care professionals. It was such an honor that she thought to ask me to prepare a small piece for their event. So, of course, I said "Yes!" and created a PowerPoint of photos taken throughout my journey, along with a forty-minute presentation for their program.

The day was remarkable, not only to see familiar faces but also to provide a patient's viewpoint. I believe it's always beneficial for medical personnel to hear from patients, so they don't lose sight of the impact they're making. I arrived early and sat in the audience, listening to the other presenters, most of whom were doctors and researchers, as I awaited my turn. I learned a lot about the process of diagnosing acute myeloid leukemia, performing bone marrow biopsies, and synthesizing all kinds of medications.

I have to admit, I began to feel overwhelmed as I sat there listening to all of these intellectuals. The doctors spewed out way too many statistics regarding the prognosis and average lifespan of survivors. My palms began to sweat. It was a bit scary for me to hear some of their findings. I believe that sometimes, when it comes to the odds of living, it's best to be kept in the dark. Having said all this, I was also grateful to be there amongst the elite. The good definitely outweighed the bad. I was even able to thank some of those who worked behind the scenes during my treatments. For instance, the doctor in charge of making my 'chemo cocktails' was there, and we briefly visited. Speaking at this conference was just the boost I needed.

Calling All Cowboys!

January was not only the month of my presentation for the healthcare providers, but also the one-year mark since my last chemo treatment! I was in a very perky mood when I showed up for my three-month routine checkup and lab work. The days have just flown by this year, and every time there is an event or holiday, I think back to the weak state I was in last year while going through chemo treatments. Everything is so different now. I imagine the newness of finally being done with CANcer will eventually fade. My hope is that forty-plus years down the road, I will still be CANcer-free and able to tell my story of miracles.

Tim came with me to this appointment, and we noticed my photo and write-up hanging on the *Faces of Hope* wall in Methodist Estabrook Cancer Center. This gallery features patients' strength and courage after having battled and conquered cancer. What an honor it was to be chosen as part of the *Faces of Hope*. It was humbling, and I pray it offers hope to others going through their CANcer journey. When I met with my doctor, he gave me encouraging news – my blood work continues to be strong. Although my platelets went down fourteen points from last time (they were 148,000 – normal range 150,000-400,000 mcL); however, he was not alarmed. I know I shouldn't worry about this, but my goal is to *stay* in the normal range. I will see my oncologist again in three months. He told me to start talking to my spleens again! It was reassuring when my doctor recognized that I could help my platelets rise through visualization, and this valuable technique was not disregarded by a medical professional. You better believe that I'll be rounding up those cowboys! Look out, spleens, here they come! Yee-haw!

Abundantly Clear

I was super excited to get a phone call from a cosmetologist at Methodist's Estabrook Inner Beauty Salon. She asked if I would be willing to model in their annual *Omaha Fashion Week – Cancer Survivor Style Show* in March. I couldn't believe it! I had never heard of this event before and, of course, took advantage of the opportunity. Yay, another thing to check off my bucket list! Who wouldn't want to be pampered like a princess? My look will be completed with nails, makeup, and hair – all styled by the best cosmetologists ever. And at the end, I'll get to walk the runway!

It feels good to be in such a healthy state of mind. It's as if the changing of the seasons to spring is heralding growth and blooming in me as well. These past few months have been full of new opportunities and experiences that I will treasure forever. I choose to capture all the opportunities around me and thank God for each of them.

Occasionally, I stop by the hospital to walk a lap in the hallway and visit with my comrades after doctor appointments. Internally, I give a salute with a smile as I pass the special room of miracles – my home away from home as I hung onto faith with each breath for several months. This hospital and the staff will always be dear to me.

I continually strive to show my children that even in adversity, we can power through. I want to be a shining light for others and give hope when fears lead us into darkness. Lately, I've been recapturing all the things to be thankful for. Shaylee and I like to tell God three things we are grateful for each day – He grants us so many blessings that we don't even realize. Having an attitude of gratitude brings a positive change in life. This attentiveness reminds me of the Bible scripture in Isaiah 43:2, "When you pass through the waters, I will be with you; and when you pass through the rivers, they will not sweep over you. When you walk through the fire, you will not be burned; the flames will not set you ablaze."

I trust that God will take care of my every step. To this day, I keep a notebook to journal blessings. It adds so much more emphasis when I reaffirm what I'm grateful for on paper. It's even fun to look back on past reflections, especially when I'm in need of some positivity. If I happen to miss a day of my journal entries, I simply continue on to the next day's date. Unless there is something extra special that I recalled from the previous day, that is. Anyone can do this. I've heard that the single best predictor of wellbeing is gratitude, and it's only a minute of your time! Make it your intention before you go to bed, or schedule any devotional time during the day. May you capture many blessings.

2 Corinthians 4:15-16 ~ All this is for your benefit, so that the grace that is reaching more and more people may cause thanksgiving to overflow to the glory of God. Therefore we do not lose heart. Though outwardly we are wasting away, yet inwardly we are being renewed day by day.

EMBRACE THE UNFAMILIARITY

It takes a lot of courage to release the familiar and seemingly secure, to embrace the new. But there is no real security in what is no longer meaningful. There is more security in the adventurous and exciting, for in movement there is life, and in change there is power.

~ Alan Cohen

Sometimes it's hard to realize the significance of a moment when you're in it. You can only see how special the experience truly was with hindsight. I've had too many of these moments to sift through, but one in particular sticks out. It happened with a colleague of mine in the summer of 2016. In mid-July, she stopped me in the hallway to tell me about a Home and Family Herbalist Program she was planning on taking. It was a two-year night class (once a week). She thought I would also be interested in taking it because of my former battle with cancer. I was very grateful for her to check with me about it and said I would give it some thought. She emailed me the initial information regarding the course outline and noted that the orientation meeting was scheduled for the following week.

I read the course syllabus and found the program intriguing. I asked Tim if he would be willing to go with me to the first meeting to hear more about it. Due to the cost and time commitment, he needed to be on board with my decision to attend. Tim agreed to go and thought that the class would be really good for me. The weekly night class was a go! There were other days to commit to during this course as well. These included a few Saturday classes involving workshops and guest speakers, lab experiences for making internal and external herbal products, and field trips. I was interested in learning about natural ways to continue with my recovery. I wanted to know how to maintain a life-long pattern of good health. If God chose to put all of these versatile plants on earth, they must be here for a reason. Herbs have healing properties like nothing else in the natural world.

The instructor of this program spent the majority of his life surrounded by herbal medicine. He also took that time to learn natural self-healing tactics, gaining plenty of survival skills in the wilderness. He is very well-rounded and has a great wealth of information. This two-year course consisted of studying ancient to modern natural herbal healing, history of eastern and western herbal medicine, principles and theory of natural healing, Native American traditions and practices, the uses of over one-hundred-fifty herbs, basics of essential oils, flower essences, aromatherapy, holistic nutrition, and so much more. I couldn't wait to venture into this new realm of medicine.

Class started this month on September 7, 2016. I look forward to our meetings each week and make sure to take ample notes. A new side of myself is beginning to blossom, and I can't wait to see where this knowledge takes me.

 2 Corinthians 9:15 ~ Thanks be to God for his indescribable gift!

FIVE

PERFECTION DOESN'T EXIST

When life doesn't go as planned, it can be discouraging. I have asked myself (more than once), "Why did this happen to me? What did I do to deserve these obstacles?" After extensive exposure to difficulty, I've begun to realize that each challenge is followed by spiritual growth. It's important to surround yourself with an environment that manifests positive transformation during challenges. I've found that reminders are one of the most helpful tools in achieving this balanced livelihood. Remind yourself to establish desired goals clearly, and set intentions for the highest good at the beginning of each day. Don't be afraid to call upon your guides, angels, archangels, or intuition for assistance at any time. Be curious about the messages you receive.

STAYING ABOVE THE WATER

We can actually be the rudder of our own mind and…
direct it where we would like it to be directed by strengthening
our capacity to voluntarily deploy our attention.

~ Richard Davidson

Let's face it – most families have a hectic life these days. If you're not rushing your children to an extracurricular activity, you're keeping up with laundry, household demands, or fixing a meal for dinner. And we can't forget about helping children with homework on top of making it to the job that pays your bills! Sometimes I wonder if it will ever be possible to set a bit of time aside for just me. Will I have to wait until the kids are out of school and on their own?

It's about time that I learn how to balance my agenda in a healthier manner. Occasionally, the everyday back-and-forth busyness makes me want to just drop everything, but I wonder how everyone would manage without me. So instead, I spend my so-called prison sentence conspiring the best time to run away and escape it all. Where would I even go? And what would I do? Visions of palm trees and massages begin to trickle in, but I know where my true obligation lies. Right now, my family needs me here.

So, unfortunately, I keep piling up the basket with tasks until it overflows. In these times of desperation, I have learned to pray to God. Simply asking for a change of scenery and just walking alone in nature can ease my mind. My break will come with time. When I return to the brimming basket in a healthier frame of mind, I sift through the overwhelming pile, perpetually searching for peace.

Don't get me wrong; I am very happy with my life. I love my family and am so blessed to be involved in everything my role as a mother consists of. Leukemia has become a distant memory, a detour that led me to my current path of life. However, on May 10, 2017, something happened that was very unexpected and left me immobile for a brief period. Let's say it was a 'wake-up' call – telling me that I need to take more time out for myself. It is necessary to rejuvenate, refill, and reflect if I want to be the best mother, daughter, wife, and friend possible. We all need breaks in life, do we not? We cannot live without taking time for intuitive rest; self-care is vital.

A while back, my appointments with my oncologist were changed from every three months to every six months. My prior consultation in November 2016 was encouraging, and my blood counts were in the normal range.

At my six-month checkup today, though, I was nervous as the nurse drew my blood for labs. I noticed a pool of blood around the needle and mentioned it to Tim because it reminded me of another time that my platelets were low. Knowing the importance of keeping your mind and heart in a positive place, I tried to brush off my anxiousness as we waited to see my doctor for the lab results. When my doctor came into the room and went over the findings of my blood work, I became distraught very quickly. My blood counts were considerably lower than they had been in the past. It was as if I briefly froze in time. This news was a complete shock because I felt fine. According to my itinerary, life was good, and everything was going as planned.

Some of my blood tests weren't finalized before Tim and I left the doctor's office. My doctor said they were just as important because it would let him know if there were any cancer "blasts" in my blood. He told me that a nurse would call when the results came in. In the meantime, a bone marrow biopsy and aspiration was set for the following day, May 11, to confirm that I am still CANcer free, God willing.

On our drive home, I received an encouraging phone call from my doctor's nurse. The blood test we were waiting for showed zero blasts – meaning there were no signs of CANcer in the blood sample, and I had a fifty-fifty chance of this being nothing. I just know I'm in the top fifty percent and have positive thoughts about this.

I debated about sharing this frightening news with family and friends because I didn't want them to worry. However, I strongly believe in the power of prayer, so I let it be known. I pray the bone marrow biopsy will show that this is just a strange happening due to the cold virus I've had for over a week. The results of the bone marrow procedure will take up to seven days. I trust in God and will keep the faith. When it comes down to it, faith is the most powerful medicine of all.

When unexpected or challenging situations occur, we are given opportunities to reflect and learn from them. What was the lesson today? I need to slow down and take time to nurture myself. Fretting over the needs of others is no longer my main priority – it is my turn to be held by Jesus.

Isaiah 41:10 ~ So do not fear, for I am with you; do not be dismayed, for I am your God. I will strengthen you and help you; I will uphold you with my righteous right hand.

Biopsy

This morning, May 11, Tim drove me to the Midwest Cancer Center in Papillion for my bone marrow biopsy and aspiration. The prayers, warm thoughts, and love sent my way from friends and family in the last twenty-four hours have meant the world to me. I have a strong feeling that my complete blood counts will balance themselves and return to normal.

When we arrived at the clinic, a nurse checked my vitals and took blood for labs. Afterward, she directed us to a small room. The nurse practitioner briefly talked about the procedure and asked me to lay on my stomach with my arms above my head. She searched my pelvic bone for a suitable location to proceed with the bone marrow biopsy and marked my skin using her fingernail imprint. After sterilizing the area, she injected it with local anesthesia to numb the region. She did a few rounds of this until reaching the bone. We waited a few minutes before proceeding.

I felt pressure and pain when the nurse practitioner struggled to get samples of my bone marrow. When she could not complete the task after a few attempts, she asked the other nurse to call for my doctor. I was so glad he was there. I took some deep breaths, wiped some tears, and repeated, "*All is well,*" as I squeezed Tim's hand tightly.

My doctor came into the room and injected more anesthesia. Tim said he made a small incision about one-quarter of an inch from where the nurse practitioner had been. He inserted a hollow needle through the bone, removed some liquid from my bone marrow, and then took a small sample of solid bone tissue. I was relieved when it was over. The nurse practitioner cleaned the area, put on a bandage, and applied pressure. After a few minutes, we were free to go.

Tim and I decided to grab lunch because I hadn't eaten much since yesterday's news. After eating, we purchased flowers to plant outdoors at our house. My doctor told me to rest for the remainder of the day, so I plan on returning to work tomorrow. Hopefully, my job will distract my mind from the vicious cycle of fearful thoughts that never seem to cease. After all, now the only thing left to do is wait. It's out of my hands for the moment.

1 Peter 5:7 ~ Cast all your anxiety on him because he cares for you.

Thy Will Be Done

 James 3:4 ~ Or take ships as an example. Although they are so large and are driven by strong winds, they are steered by a very small rudder wherever the pilot wants to go.

The dictionary describes the word journey as "something suggesting travel from one place to another." Well, I have been to many places on my CANcer journey; and I seem to be entering into another part – waiting to find out if my leukemia has returned. Once again, I feel as if I am in uncharted territory. However, God has healed me in the past. He is my pilot and compass, and I will need His guidance to direct my next course of action. Even though I feel and know – with all my heart and soul – this challenging time will pass, I am still experiencing MANY emotions.

For the past week or so, I have been leaning on techniques learned throughout my past CANcer experience. I remembered that visualization is very impactful and pictured myself going through stored files (if you will) in my brain to help this situation go more smoothly. I visualized myself in a place that is very sacred to me – a place where I feel serenity, tranquility, pure joy, and have good health. Visualization is a powerful healing tool; you don't need to physically go to your sacred place to feel its effect. You only need to picture it in your mind. So, this is what I did to ease my nerves.

I also found comfort by wrapping myself in my prayer shawl from time to time this week. In addition, I went to the computer and typed the specific number range I wanted my complete blood count (CBC) to be. I made six copies and taped each to various locations in my home (one in my vehicle), so I would notice them and manifest these changes in my body coming to fruition.

My hope has remained high with every turn, even though fear has also been with me. Sometimes, waiting for results makes me feel more uneasy than just hearing them right away. In the afternoon of May 15, I received a call from my doctor at the Methodist Estabrook Cancer Center. He said that I had a recurrence of acute myeloid leukemia. The preliminary tests showed forty percent blasts in my bone marrow, and I needed to meet with him on May 16, to go over the next steps. My doctor said the final results would be coming within the next couple of days. I asked if there was a chance that the final test results would come back in my favor. He told me that that chance was slim, but I still had hope.

This part of my journey began with shock – my CBC's were not consistent with past readings, and suddenly my life was in danger again. After my doctor told me about the cancer's return, I was consumed with fear of the unknown and began questioning my every move these past six months, attempting to point a finger at whatever may have caused it. Was it because I had a small electric shock from my diffuser? Was it due to a two-week cleanse that I recently completed? Have I been too hard on my body? Was it this, was it that? The list goes on and on. And when I finally realized the seal on my fate, there were tears. I prayed to God that nothing but good would come out of this situation – perhaps He still had lessons for me to learn. I take comfort in a verse from Joshua 1:9, "Have I not commanded you? Be strong and courageous. Do not be afraid; do not be discouraged, for the LORD your God will be with you wherever you go."

Since last week, all of my children have been alerted about what was going on. After hearing the final results, we sat together as a family and told them what the doctor said. We feel it's important to be upfront about my health. I assured my kids that I would fight with everything in me to get through this again. I choose life and will continue to move forward with faith, hope, and determination.

We went to my parents' house, and I just sobbed in my mother's arms. Knowing that I had to compete for my life once again was terrifying. Memories of the jagged cliffs I needed to climb over to get healthy last time began swirling through my mind. How am I going to get through this again? It was in the depths of this sorrow that I was reminded of a quote by John Green, "The darkest nights produce the brightest stars." And I shifted my attention back to HOPE.

 Hebrews 11:1 ~ Now faith is confidence in what we hope for and assurance about what we do not see.

G.I. Mary Jane Returns!

At my appointment on May 16, my doctor told us the next steps. This time, unlike the last, I need to have a stem cell transplant from a donor if I want long-term survival and a cure. Furthermore, I will need to leave my current oncologist and hospital family (whom I loved and trusted) and join a new one that has a facility fit for allogeneic (donor) stem cell transplants. Matt will need to be tested right away to see if he is a compatible donor. There is a twenty-five percent chance of him being a match. If he is not suitable, we need to look nationwide for a perfect fit. I have hope that it will all work out.

While we are searching for a donor, I will get chemotherapy treatments, like last time (induction phase), to reach remission. Once in remission, I may need an additional round of chemo (consolidation phase) to keep me that way. Then, I will go through another round of intense chemo for six days to bring my blood counts down to zero, with blood and platelet transfusions as needed to sustain my life. Finally, after all that preparation, comes the stem cell transplant. The first one hundred days are critical. I must stay healthy during that time because it takes a while for my immune system to reboot and fight off infections. Additionally, I might need to take lifelong medication to ensure my body never rejects the transplanted stem cells.

If all goes well, I will be healthy and live a long life, never having to worry about CANcer again. My doctor said this is just bad luck, and there is nothing I could have done to stop it. My stem cells have a glitch. He said it just happened, and we need to move forward by not feeling guilty or guessing why. It made me feel better knowing that there was nothing I could have done to prevent this relapse. As I wipe my tears away, I've decided that G.I. Mary Jane is ready for battle – I will once again kick CANcer's butt! My COURAGE, FAITH, and HOPE stand at the ready.

 John 14:27 ~ Peace I leave with you; my peace I give you. I do not give to you as the world gives. Do not let your hearts be troubled and do not be afraid.

FIRST IMPRESSIONS

Almost everyone will make a good first impression,
but only a few will make a good lasting impression.

~ Sonja Parker

There's something to be said about making a positive first impression. It leaves a lasting effect when you are welcomed with a friendly smile and buoyant demeanor. Anyone can make an initial encounter meaningful, but not everyone has the personality to make it memorable. I'm pleased that my first impression at Nebraska Medicine on May 18, was remarkable. Just two days after finding out about the recurrence of leukemia, I met with my new hematologist/oncologist, who specializes in stem cell transplants. It's imperative to move fast when tackling leukemia, not to mention a relapse. Doctors don't know precisely how or when drastic changes can happen for the worse if not treated with chemotherapy right away. My current doctor, whom I've grown to trust over the past two and a half years, will now be in the peripheral as I make my way into another frightening unknown. All I can do now is pray for a brave spirit and the best outcome.

Upon arrival at the large Nebraska Medicine facility, we found our way to my new doctor's suite, where a group of individuals dressed in Hawaiian attire greeted us (lei's, grass skirts, flower bandanas, and coconut bras). They had many colored lei's draped over their arms and asked, "Do you want to get lei'd?" I said, "Well, of course!" They shouted, "All right!" and picked out a coral/orange-colored lei for me to wear. Little did they know that this happened to be similar to the ribbon color of leukemia. As Tim was handed a lei too, I couldn't resist saying to one of the guys, "I like your coconuts!" They all laughed, and we asked them if they came to the office often – a little chemo humor goes a long way! Through our conversation, we found out that it was the last day of chemo for one of the men in the group, and they were celebrating. It was so much fun to visit with them, and I feel God put me there at that time to ease my nerves and give me hope for the future.

Shortly after that, we met a nurse who would be my case manager. She gave Tim and me a lot of information about stem cell transplants and a list of resources. When the doctor came in, he took his time with us and answered all our questions. Most importantly, he assured me that I could survive this illness yet another time. I appreciated that he asked us to tell him about ourselves and genuinely seemed interested in what we had to say. I told him that I was a fighter – determined to survive for the sake of my family.

We discussed options for the first phase of treatment (induction phase). My doctor recommended using the same seven-day/three-day chemo cocktail as last time. That's a twenty-four-hour drip of chemo for seven days, with an additional type of chemo on the first three days and only the primary type for the remainder of the week. A few days after finishing this treatment, I need another bone marrow biopsy to confirm I've reached remission. Once in remission, we will move forward with the stem cell transplant, which includes chemotherapy cocktails of even greater potency.

Currently, we are waiting for insurance approval so that Nebraska Medicine can mail my brother, Matt, the supplies needed to test for a match. These chemo treatments will be for nothing if we can't find a suitable stem cell donor. The test is easy – Matt simply has to swab the inside of his cheek and send it back through priority mail. The results take about two weeks. If he is a match, we will be thrilled! If not, my sixteen-year-old son, Brody, will be tested. From there, we will look nationwide. Our last resort would be worldwide. When I asked Brody if he would consider it, he did not hesitate for one second and said, "Of course, why wouldn't I? You're my mom!" Wow, what a brave young man I have!

With this relapse, I was given the choice of having my induction phase of treatments at Methodist Hospital (as before) or starting fresh with Nebraska Medicine. Either way, I would have the stem cell transplant at Nebraska Medicine. We were told to call them later in the day with our decision.

Tim and I thought long and hard about which facility would be best for the induction phase. This decision was difficult because I had the best experience at Methodist and already formed relationships with so many, not to mention the excellent rapport I already had with my oncologist. However, I decided to make an abrupt switch in my medical care team and fully commit to Nebraska Medicine. I wanted a chance to connect with their healthcare system, which would ultimately be taking care of me during my stem cell transplant. Not only did I feel it was vital for the medical care team to know my character, but I also needed to get a feel for the individuals who held my life in their hands. I wanted the medical care team to know me and understand the lengths I was willing to go for survival.

My new doctor wanted me to start chemo right away. So, I finished up a few things at work the following morning, May 19, and was admitted to Nebraska Medicine that afternoon to begin treatments. Three nurses came to put in a PICC line (like last time). A short while later, the pharmacist introduced herself. I asked about using essential oils and natural herbs throughout this process, as both are very important to me. The pharmacist wrote down the herbal regimen and essential oils I wanted to use. She was hesitant to let me use any of it, which was very discouraging. She said she would follow up with me after researching how the natural medicine would react with the chemo cocktail and other medications.

Tim and I also had a visit from the chaplain. It was a very busy day. Later, I found out that I could not take herbs while in the hospital and was only approved to use three of the several essential oils that I brought with me. However, even with these restrictions, my medical care team allowed me to use my herbal remedies and essential oils when I was not actively undergoing treatment at the hospital. The moment I was discharged, I returned to natural medicine, as my herbalist recommended. Balancing eastern and western medicine felt like the only way for me to heal as quickly as possible; my compromise with the medical staff was greatly appreciated.

I often wonder if Reiki was another healing modality that helped me through the darkest days of my previous CANcer journey. Even though I didn't utilize its potential healing power nearly as much as I could have, I am confident that universal energy was a key factor in my rejuvenation. At that time, I was more open to other friends sending me healing energy rather than doing it myself. I was under the impression that their skills would work better than my own. Back then, Reiki wasn't something I used daily, and I was unsure of my abilities. It was a behind-the-scenes addition to my toolbox of wellbeing ideas.

Perhaps Reiki worked naturally, though, because it was ingrained into my core. I'd like to believe that's the case. Everyone has the ability to focus energy when their intentions are pure. The trick is to allow the energy to do the work – it will flow where it needs to go. The Reiki practitioner is merely the conduit for the energy flow.

Interestingly enough, just days before my doctor's appointment earlier this month, I had a Level Two Reiki attunement from the same woman I met in the *A Time to Heal* class. It had been nearly a year since the Level One Reiki attunement, and my interest had grown considerably since then. After all, her suggestion of using visualization to raise my platelets worked, and I was fascinated to learn more about healing energy. I had just finished reading a self-help Reiki book and wrote down questions as they arose so I wouldn't forget to ask them during our time together. It was perfect timing because the newly found recurrence was literally just days after I met with her.

It was as if God put the desire in my heart to learn more about Reiki and complete Level Two, even though I don't talk about it outside of my home. I have been worried about how my parents and friends would react to energy work because of their lack of knowledge surrounding it. My parents seemed hesitant about this healing modality because they didn't know if it was a Christian method. Therefore, I mostly kept my learnings to myself or within my home, amongst Tim and our children. I didn't want to pressure anyone into my new way of thinking or push them away because of my new interest. It wasn't until much later that my parents opened up to the idea of Reiki. Over time, they have grown accustomed to my use of energy work and now love the positive effects that it harbors! It's fascinating what a bit of open-mindedness can do.

 Ephesians 6:10 ~ Finally, be strong in the Lord and in his mighty power.

SIX

PROOF OF LIFE

Conflict and stress can fracture our lives. These fractures, if occurring too quickly and appearing too close together, are capable of breaking us completely; however, no suffering is too great to be healed. Each crack creates openings for the light of love to shine through. A trial of sorrow makes way for the brightest pleasure. Love heals all.

BE THE MATCH

Anyone can give up, it's the easiest thing in the world to do.
But to hold it together when everyone else would understand
if you fell apart, that's true strength.

~ Unknown

When my doctor informed me that I had a recurrence of acute myeloid leukemia and needed a stem cell transplant for long-term survival, I was terrified. Even so, I still had my faith. Many family and friends have contacted me about their willingness to be a stem cell donor, and I sincerely appreciate their thoughtfulness. But time is waning, and my doctor needs to take the necessary steps quickly for my best outcome. For insurance to cover the costs of this transplant (ten to fifteen thousand dollars to test just one person), we have to follow a very specific protocol. Some insurances put a cap on how many people can be tested for a match. God-willing, my brother will be my match. Matt might be the best chance I have.

I learned an interesting fact: If my stem cell transplant comes from a male, my DNA will accept the male XY chromosomes. Instead of having the women's XX chromosomes, mine will be XY for the rest of my life – this means a bone marrow biopsy will show that I'm a man! After hearing this, I just chuckled and told my doctor, "As long as I don't grow a beard and testicles, I can handle that!" But inside, I was scared of what life would be like after the transplant — if I would be one of the lucky patients to survive such an intense procedure, that is. And what kind of residual, long-lasting side effects was I going to experience? I did my best to hide my fears with humor, but I've had moments of tears behind closed doors. I have privately poured out my emotions during meditative prayers, short walks, or during quiet moments with Tim.

Matt anxiously awaited the swab kit's arrival so he could be tested before we had to search nationwide. Fingers crossed that he's in the twenty-five percent group of matched siblings. Matt and I had a good laugh when he said he was going to start eating healthier and working out to get ready for this, just in case he was my perfect match. While his intentions are good, I'm not sure if a few weeks of diet and exercise would make a huge difference. I know he wants the best for me, though, and I love him so much for that. I often wonder how he *really* feels about being my potential donor. Does he have the same fears as I do? How would he feel if the transplant didn't work? And would that lead to guilt? I certainly hope not. Honestly, we haven't talked about these things. I guess we all have just been doing our best to stay positive and make it through each day.

The medical care team also wanted to test my oldest son, Brody. He had an appointment with my case manager the other day. She went over the stem cell transplant process and explained that sometimes patients don't survive. If this should be the case for me, she wanted Brody to understand that it would not be his fault. A counselor was also there for this conversation. I'm sure this was very difficult for a sixteen-year-old to hear. After the meeting, Brody came to my hospital room. I talked to him about the test and assured him that he did not need to take on this responsibility for my sake. I knew it would be an enormous burden to bear, especially at his young age, should something not go as expected. Brody never once hesitated, though. He told me that he would do anything for me. It was the most humbling, loving gift I could ever ask for – my son as my donor, if it was God's will.

At this time, the plan is to use Matt's stem cells if he is the best match. If not, Brody is next in line. No matter what, I trust that my doctor will find a suitable donor, even if the search ends up being nationwide or worldwide. I am doing my best to prepare for this long process. It seems like everything around me is moving in slow motion, and I have no control over space and time. Up until now, I've known what to expect from the cancer healing process. I'm familiar with the side effects of chemo because I've already been through it once – this stem cell transplant is a whole new ball game, and I have every intention to win.

During one of these slow-moving moments, I started thinking about when I played softball as a pitcher and catcher while growing up. I always had a love for the game. My secret weapon was that I was left-handed. When it was my turn to bat, I could see the pitcher's sudden loss of confidence as I stepped up to the plate. It was a known fact that left-handers were difficult to pitch to, and it was common for them to walk to first base due to poor throws and not clearing the strike zone.

Every player has an important job when they're on the field, but if the pitcher freezes and makes errors, the defending team has the potential to make it to home plate much more easily. The stress level can quickly accelerate when pitches don't fall in the strike zone and the batter walks to first base. Sometimes this anxiousness causes the pitcher to choke and continue walking batters for the rest of the inning or until the coach switches the pitcher out. This dismissal happened to me on occasion, and when it did, my coach ordered me to sit on the bench for the rest of the inning. It was a bit embarrassing, but at the same time, I was relieved that the pressure was taken off me. It was nice not to worry about letting my team down even more.

We all need to take breaks to collect our thoughts and regain our stability. When I was playing softball, I learned that it was beneficial for me to sit on the bench when my pitching wasn't on target. I would take a few deep breaths, recenter, and refuel my confidence while waiting for the next inning. It's funny how these memories flood back to the surface at the oddest times. While I sit here waiting for my match, I am comforted that these past experiences came to me for a reason. At this point, I'm in the midst of my own 'softball' tournament, only this time, the 'victory' of life is much more permanent. I can picture it now, it's the last inning, and I am up to bat for the winning score. I imagine myself receiving the perfect pitch and knocking the ball out of the park. With great anticipation and confidence, I steadily jog to first base, then second and third, until safely completing my home run of perfect wellness. Fans roar in the stands with excitement, lifting me up with their prayers and praises.

The message of my memory was that sometimes we need to take a step back until we know we are ready to perform our best. Defeating CANcer is all about patience, and as long as I keep up the morale, I CAN overcome it. I'm ready to get back into the game and achieve the greatest victory of all.

 Philippians 4:19-20 ~ And my God will meet all your needs according to the riches of his glory in Christ Jesus. To our God and Father be glory for ever and ever. Amen.

SONG OF PRAISE

There are things known and there are things unknown,
and in between are the doors of perception.

~ Aldous Huxley

Custodians are the backbones of commercial buildings and often don't get enough credit for what they do. Cleanliness is crucial for me right now, and all of their sanitizing makes me feel more secure. Recently, I was blessed to visit with a custodian who cleans patients' rooms. She has a radiant smile and a tranquil aura about her. A few years ago, this woman migrated to the United States from West Africa to give her children a better life. She asked if she could sing to me as I laid sluggishly in bed. I was pleasantly surprised by her request and welcomed it. She sang "How Great Thou Art" as she mopped the floor. The touching verses somehow lifted the heaviness off my shoulders. I thanked her for the heartfelt song of praise. She often comes into my room with worship hymns, revitalizing my spirit with her radiant voice. God is in ALL the details once again.

The other day, the Chaplain brought me an unexpected gift – a prayer shawl. I love my visits with the Chaplain (just as I did at Methodist). When she comes, we pray, she gives me communion, and she anoints me. When she brought me the shawl, she explained that she searched and searched for the ideal one with no luck. It was only after looking in a completely separate cupboard that she found the perfect shawl for me. It's a delightful knitted rainbow of pastel colors. I told her about my 'rainbows' and how they were a sign that God was with me. She had known nothing about the significance rainbows held in my heart when she was picking out this magical shawl. I am surrounded by lovely people here at Nebraska Medicine.

Life is such a mystery. We move through it in ignorance, trying to keep our eyes open. And when we can't find the answer, we search frantically for some immediate solution. It's sad that some people won't admit they need help until a crisis arrives. True growth can only be achieved when we realize that help is always there. We need to blindly have faith that God will show us the way in every circumstance.

Colossians 3:17 ~ And whatever you do, whether in word or deed, do it all in the name of the Lord Jesus, giving thanks to God the Father through Him.

NEWFOUND INDEPENDENCE

Between stimulus and response, there is a space.
In that space is our power to choose our response.
In our response lies our growth and our freedom.

~ Vicktor E. Frankl

It's May 27 – a brand new day! Late last night, I finally broke free from the constraints of my companion Roly (AKA: chemo cart). It is such a great feeling not to be tied down, and of course, to have made it through the seven-day treatment. No more dragging the chemo cart here and there or struggling to complete simple tasks like showering or even using the restroom. Over the past seven days, my sidekick has reminded me of the value of independence. I'm sure others remember a time when a boyfriend or girlfriend smothered them by never leaving their side, as if they were attached at the hip and couldn't break loose. Sometimes this attachment can leave us feeling powerless. I should be grateful, though. At least Roly doesn't talk back or disagree with me!

Ultimately, we all need some time to ourselves. I'm realizing now more than ever that I need to opt out of dependent shenanigans. Tim and the kids are doing just fine without me managing appointments, practices, and housework. Tim has already started paying Holly to take care of the laundry duties. He proudly says, "She is on top of it too!" The other kids complete miscellaneous chores, and he pays them what he thinks the job is worth. It's sad to admit, but money talks at this age. Maybe I'll come home to a new set of well-rounded kids! They've always had weekly chores, but the list has gotten quite a bit longer – and I think it's good for them to help around the house more. It builds character.

Speaking of character, G.I. Mary Jane is back kickin' CANcer's butt one day at a time! Yesterday, I got the BIG head shave and felt badder than ever!

Failure is not an option! I look forward to breaking out of this joint within the next couple of weeks and reuniting with my family at home.

 Colossians 3:12 ~ Therefore, as God's chosen people, holy and dearly loved, clothe yourselves with compassion, kindness, humility, gentleness, and patience.

FRED & PAMELA BUFFETT CANCER CENTER OPEN HOUSE

Each time we face our fear, we gain strength, courage, and confidence in the doing.

~ Theodore Roosevelt

Initially, I decided NOT to walk through the Fred & Pamela Buffett Cancer Center's Open House on May 27, even though I could because I wasn't hooked up to the chemo cart anymore. But a woman has every right to change her mind! Sometimes, I overanalyze situations in my head before determining the best option, even for the simplest tasks. For example, if Tim asks, "Do you want to go out to eat?" I say, "It depends on where you're thinking about going." The conversation goes back and forth with, "What are you in the mood for?" "I don't know. What do you want?" These back and forth questions continue until one of us makes a final decision. Sometimes it's just easier to stay home, especially when the kids also want to be involved in the decision-making process. The same goes with which pair of footwear looks best with the outfit I'm wearing on any given day. Most mornings, I ask Holly or Shaylee which option most fits with the attire – this pair or that. After the girls state their opinions, I usually go with my gut reaction anyway.

When I stop to reflect upon this, it's rather comical, and I'm sure the girls grow weary of me, but they still add their two cents worth. Maybe it's not their advice I seek, but rather a confirmation that I had made the right choice in the first place. Seeking validation is something that women, or at least I, do all the time. It's almost as if we think we need to ask permission before sharing our wants, needs, and opinions. This uncertainty is likely due to the sad truth that we will be immediately shut down if we say the wrong thing. Men often don't take us seriously in politics, the workforce, or business exchanges. Additionally, the media (ads, fashion industry, magazines, movies, and so on) conditions us NOT to trust ourselves but to trust society instead. One wrong move feels detrimental, so sometimes I wonder if it's easier not to make any moves at all.

This grueling process of overthinking is how I would have made the final decision to go to the open house, but I ran into a lady in the hallway that made the answer clear. She had just come from the open house and described it as absolutely stunning. She was going to see if her sister was up for a wheelchair ride through the beautiful scenery and asked if I would like to join them. It was decision time – I needed to respond quickly to avoid missing the opportunity to go. Up until that moment, I had decided not to go due to public exposure, but now the idea of walking with someone by my side in this daunting endeavor made it seem doable, enjoyable even! I asked my nurse, and it was approved, but only if I wore gloves and a mask. I quickly grabbed my phone so that I could take pictures. My new friends and I were prepared to tackle any challenge that came our way. I knew she would make sure her sister and I didn't have to touch anything, such as elevator buttons.

Our protector pushed her sister in the wheelchair, and I strolled alongside them. We gazed at all the beautiful artwork and Chihuly glass-blown pieces displayed throughout the quarters. The open house was spread throughout several different areas and floors – and we explored them all! This brief escapade energized me, and the sunlight on my face reminded me of the peace we can find in happiness. The entire trip filled my heart with joy and left quite an impression. I was glad I changed my mind and went with them.

When I returned to my room, the nurses gave me a change of clothes, and I showered. The adventure was well worth it. I can't wait to move to the Fred & Pamela Buffett Cancer Center on June 6. The colored fragments of light shining through the decorative glass-blown structures confirmed that this is a place of healing.

John 14:27 ~ Peace I leave with you; my peace I give you. I do not give to you as the world gives. Do not let your hearts be troubled and do not be afraid.

SHAWL OF GOD'S HEALING ARMS

*Rest. Allow God to restore, replenish
and refocus your heart and mind.*

~ Unknown

May 28, came with some strange happenings, including a miracle! I woke up feeling slightly different than I had in the past few days. I just felt a little off – not necessarily light-headed, but faint. I proceeded to eat breakfast and shower. After visiting with the doctor and hearing that I needed a platelet transfusion because my platelets were at 10,000 (normal range 150,000-400,000 mcL), I went for a walk in the halls. Maybe some movement would make me feel better.

On my walk, I noticed that I was moving at a much slower pace than usual. That didn't bother me, but I knew something was not right. After a few more rounds in the hall, I ran into my new friend. We've frequently been visiting since my admittance into Nebraska Medicine on May 19. Her nineteen-year-old son is currently battling acute myeloid leukemia (AML). This is his third battle with cancer; he had Hodgkin's Lymphoma at the age of sixteen and experienced a relapse shortly after reaching remission. He had used his own stem cells (autologous stem cell transplant) to tackle Hodgkin's Lymphoma for good. Even with this victory, however, there was a 2-percent chance of him contracting AML from the chemo they used to treat his type of cancer. Sadly, he was in this 2 percent group.

While we were in the hall visiting, his mom shared how upset she was about his negative attitude. She mentioned that he was depressed, very angry (at the world and God), and wanted to go home. He told her that he'd rather die than go through cancer again. Recently, the chemo put his AML in remission, and he is currently recovering. His doctor is preparing for a donor-based stem cell transplant as we speak. He's already halfway there, and I know he can do this! My heart breaks for his mother, though.

I wish he would give me a chance to visit with him, but he clearly doesn't want to talk to me, and I don't want to press the issue. Honestly, I don't know that I would be helpful anyway.

All of a sudden, as his mother was talking, I got clammy and could feel sweat beads accumulate on my forehead. Things got a little blurry, and I told her that I needed to keep walking. She asked if I was all right as a nurse rushed over. I said I felt like I was going to faint. A rolling chair was next to us, and I sat down. The nurse immediately wheeled me to my room and helped me to bed. The faint feeling diminished as fast as it came, but it was a bit scary for me. My doctor said we would check for low blood sugar levels if it happens again.

Fortunately, my donor's platelets arrived as all the excitement was happening, so the nurses gave me Benadryl to help prevent a reaction before receiving them. The initial transfusion went well, but complications started plaguing me within about twenty minutes. I was almost asleep when suddenly my body began shaking vigorously from chills. I waited for a short while, hoping they would go away, but then my muscles began to ache. So, I called the tech to request a warm blanket. She came right away, and I waited another ten minutes. With no relief from the chills, I called the tech again and requested another warm blanket.

'Prayer shawl' came to my mind, so I asked her to please bring me the prayer shawl that Holly's piano teacher gave me three years ago. It is alive with the Holy Spirit – God wraps me in His loving arms whenever I wear it. This prayer shawl is a witness to countless miracles. And, sure enough, when the nurse lifted it off the couch and placed it on my body, the all-powerful spirit of that wrap ceased my chills in minutes! The comfort of my prayer shawl granted me a few hours of peaceful sleep. After all my miracles, I know now that the shawl alone is not my savior. The Spirit of God within the shawl is what I must be thankful for. The next day was a day of rest for my weary soul.

 Genesis 2:1-2 ~ Thus the heavens and the earth were completed in all their vast array. By the seventh day God had finished the work he had been doing; so on the seventh day he rested from all his work.

COURAGE UNDER FIRE

*When we learn how to become resilient, we learn how to
embrace the beautifully broad spectrum of the human experience.*

~ Jaeda DeWalt

It has been three days since the Fred & Pamela Buffett Cancer Center's
Open House, and I was thrilled to hear that I could travel through it once
more. I had to get permission to leave the floor just as last time, but they
let me go as long as I promised to keep my mask and gloves on. A friend
of mine was visiting at the time, and she pushed me in the wheelchair
because I was too weak to make the long trek in my current state. It was so
wonderful to see all the beautiful glass-blown artwork again. She took me
outside to the Healing Garden, and I was reminded of how comforting the
heat of the sun can be. I can't wait to move into this new building.

The next day, Tim and Colby came to visit. Tim always has a few jokes
for the nurses, and we have a lot of laughs. Just as the saying goes, "Laughter
is the best medicine!" We were also permitted to go to the new Buffett
Center, and Colby enjoyed pushing me in the wheelchair. I don't think
patients could ever get tired of seeing that place. Words can't adequately
describe its glory. I can tell that a great deal of research, time, and money
was put into its design.

That afternoon, my doctor scheduled a bone marrow biopsy and
aspiration to determine if the intense chemo regimen had successfully put me
in remission. I've had many bone marrow biopsies, but June 1, was a 'bone
marrow biopsy gone bad' day. Nebraska Medicine does them differently
than I've ever seen before. I lay on my stomach, as usual. They use the same
numbing agent (that stings), then go into the pelvic bone and collect bone
marrow (aspiration) with a hollow needle attached to an electric hand drill
to collect the bone sample. I tolerated everything until the electric drill. The
nurse practitioner accidentally drilled through my entire bone, and I could
feel the flesh inside my body shred as my leg automatically reacted with a
jerk. She must have caught some nerve endings. It was a terrible experience
that Tim and Colby shouldn't have witnessed.

I sobbed for a few minutes but tried to hold my emotions inside for Tim and Colby's sake. The nurse practitioner said that she didn't mean to go in that far. Apparently, there are markers on the needle to let them know how far to go in, but she said that since I'm petite, the indicators weren't as accurate. After the practitioner banged the needle on the table several times (because there was so much bone in the hollow needle), she was able to get the bone out and showed all of us the bone sample. It was a very long piece of bone. I asked her if there were any organs that she could have nicked with the drill. She said it was just meat (or muscle) and that I shouldn't worry about it. But I *was* worried – this accidental mishap could have detrimental consequences. I was concerned that something terrible might come from it. I began to pray for proper healing in Jesus' name! I was desperate for another miracle, another sign that God was with me. At this moment, that was the only thing keeping me together.

When I finally calmed down, I glanced at the cart next to my hospital bed and noticed my devotional books and scriptures. I decided to read that day's devotion from *Jesus Calling* by Sarah Young. Three sentences really resonated with me, "Expect to find trouble in this day. At the same time, trust that *My way is perfect*, even in the midst of such messy imperfection. Stay conscious of Me as you go through this day, remembering that I never leave your side." Tears of relief rolled down my cheeks, and I thanked God for showing me that He was, is, and will forever be with me – even on the most challenging of days. This devotion gave me the reassurance I needed. I was in pain, uncertain, and scared because I didn't know if this would negatively affect my overall recovery. I didn't have the immune system to ward off infections or injuries induced by the bone marrow biopsy. My loved ones did all they could to soothe me, but it was the Word of God that ultimately came through. The trauma of this experience will not stop me from reaching my goals. I pray for the strength of Samson and the patience of Job as I finish destroying this cancer.

 Psalm 50:15 ~ Then call on me when you are in trouble, and I will rescue you, and you will give me glory.

Preliminary results are in!

 Psalm 30:2 ~ LORD my God, I called to you for help, and you healed me.

The bone marrow biopsy confirmed that the chemo treatments were successful and that I'm in remission. Immediately after hearing this fantastic news, I took a winner's lap in the hospital's hallway to celebrate. This development means it's time to move faster and find a suitable donor for my stem cell transplant. We discovered that my brother was not a good match, and after several blood tests, neither was my son, Brody. *Be The Match* began its search nationwide for the perfect donor. Hopefully they find that person quickly!

While on my walk, a man I've noticed in my peripheral for the past few days stopped me and said, "I know you're a fighter. You will get through this. You have that spark in your eyes, and it shows." He went on to say that he was glad to have told me this before he left the hospital. His wife had been battling cancer for a while, and they were getting ready to go home on hospice. It was sad to see them leave, and I told him that I would be praying for their family as they go through this process. We never know when God will call us home, but we do know that God will be there with arms wide open when it happens. I know there is life after death on Earth – an abundance of love, peace, and pure joy.

 Hebrews 11:1 ~ Now faith is confidence in what we hope for and assurance about what we do not see.

THE BIG MOVE: A PLACE OF HEALING

I go to nature to be soothed, and healed,
and to have my senses put in order.

~ John Burroughs

I can't believe today is my last full day in the old section of the hospital. Tim and my dad came to pack up all my belongings so that I would be ready for the BIG move to the new Fred & Pamela Buffett Cancer Center tomorrow, June 6. My energy is limited, so their assistance was so appreciated. The past couple of days has been busy with blood and platelet transfusions. I've come to recognize that my body tells me when I need blood by giving me a pulsating headache. Once the blood transfusion is complete, my headache goes away. I told the nurses that my brain communicates with me when it needs more oxygen!

It's so interesting that our bodies can reveal our needs through pain, discomfort, or even pleasure. We just need to become more in-tune with what our body is trying to tell us. For instance, if I am anxious, stressed, or hesitant about something and my stomach is in knots with just the thought of it, I take more time to ponder on the idea to see if it resonates with me and is the correct choice. It's also helpful to talk through concerns with a trusted friend or ask questions when you don't fully understand what the situation entails.

On the other hand, when I feel at ease or have a calm sensation flow through me, I trust that my decision has my wellbeing in mind. I like to think of this as my intuition or gut-feeling kicking in. I've come to realize that when it comes down to it, I am the only one who looks out for my best interest. I am in charge of my life and emotions. Physical cues give us chances to control the outcomes of our lives. So, whenever a headache makes an appearance these days, I will always question if I need a transfusion.

This particular day seemed to go by quickly. Most likely because having family by my side always has a way of lifting my spirits. When Tim and my parents left, I walked a few more laps in the hallway, brushed my teeth, and got settled into bed for the night. After I had been sleeping for a while, the tech took my temperature (as it's routinely done every few hours), and it was 101.4 degrees. The nurse said they might need to do cultures again. My heart sank, and I told her that I had just gotten too warm under my covers. Immediately, I took off my covers and fanned my legs back and forth. I asked if they would retake my temperature. They agreed to do it doubtingly, and it was 99.1 degrees – what a miracle! Both of them couldn't believe it and had never seen anything like that happen before. I told them it was God! The nurse said, "Now I really do believe in miracles!" I fell back to sleep, dreaming of my new room. In a few short hours, I'll be peering through the window at all the beautiful scenery – very different from the brick-building view across my current room. There will be so much more light and love in the space.

Tim, Brody, and Shaylee came very early in the morning to be with me for the BIG move, helping me get everything situated in the new cancer center. A Nebraska Medicine representative came in to ask if they could film me going to my room and get a quick interview afterward. I was honored to be asked and said, "Of course!"

The tech wheeled me to the entrance of the Fred & Pamela Buffett Cancer Center, and then I walked down the long hallway. Many nurses and techs were greeting me. In the distance, I saw Tim, Brody, and Shaylee walking toward me. It was a joyous welcome. The walls were brightly colored and made me feel more alive. When I entered my room and saw the natural light flowing through, my heart danced with excitement. Everything was perfect! It was such an inspiring, hope-filled place to heal. The entire facility is decked with unbelievable works of art, uniting love and healing with creative expression.

As I looked around the room, I noticed Tim and the kids had all my belongings in order. Our family pictures and Shaylee's artwork were on full display. The dreadful brick building no longer blocked the view from my window, and I was blessed with several hours of direct sunlight per day. I looked outside to discover a fantastic vision of the Healing Garden below, plus speckles of trees in the distance. I couldn't have been more pleased. This place was surreal. At that point, the only thing I needed to do was continue building strength for the stem cell transplant.

Psalm 23:1-4 ~ The LORD is my shepherd, I lack nothing. He makes me lie down in green pastures, he leads me beside quiet waters, he refreshes my soul. He guides me along the right paths for his name's sake. Even though I walk through the darkest valley, I will fear no evil, for you are with me; your rod and your staff, they comfort me.

There's No Place Like Home

I've been in the Fred & Pamela Buffett Cancer Center for two days and already feel more life in my body. It's as if every part of me – every cell – is being individually revitalized. On top of the natural light and beautiful scenery, there are several new locations for me to roam around. The release from being confined to tight quarters is so sweet. I even have opportunities to go outdoors and get fresh air if I wear a mask.

On June 7, Tim, Holly, Colby, and I were sitting at the water feature in the Healing Garden when a doctor came toward us. It was the same physician I had seen that morning. He sat next to me and said he had good news. They were going to stop my IV antibiotic and monitor how I do with the oral antibiotic throughout the day and night. If my temperature remained stable overnight, they were going to let me go home for a couple of weeks. I was thrilled, but a part of me knew that my immune system was literally zero right now. They feel that I will be fine at home with proper handwashing and the use of masks/gloves until my blood counts rise. I need to remind myself that I got through this before and will do the same again.

The night went beautifully. No fevers! However, I do tend to wake up in the middle of the night wet (soaked) with sweat. Sometimes, I need to change my gown due to its dampness. My body has been through a lot and is working hard to normalize. I recall this happening all too well during my prior recovery in 2014.

The familiar drive home was captivating. I had missed the green crops surrounding our neighborhood. When I stepped into my house, the kids were anxiously awaiting my arrival and greeted me like a queen! They often ask if I need anything and take good care of me. Of course, Tim does an excellent job at this too. They had worked so hard dusting everything, including the ceiling fans, getting new filters for our air purifiers, and cleaning the entire house. I appreciated everything my family did to avoid complications while my blood counts rose.

Shortly after we arrived home in the early evening of June 8, I put on a mask and gloves to walk briefly outdoors. Since I live in the country, the doctor told me that I need to be extra cautious outside due to the excess pollen and dust from farmland, trees, and flowers. There is a possibility of fungal spores or mold getting into my lungs. It's not worth the risk to me. I also need to wear a mask and gloves anytime I go to the hospital for blood products until my counts rise to an adequate level on their own. During my walk, I enjoyed hearing the birds chirp around me and seeing the leaves blow gently in the breeze. My dog, Rick, followed me around and protected me from any harm. Even though my walk was slow and brief, it was refreshing to be outdoors.

Still Searching for a Match

Since we recently found out that Brody is not my best match. *Be The Match* has made contact with two of five potential ten-of-ten matches and will continue to try to reach the other three. In the meantime, these two men scheduled appointments for more blood work this week because my doctors needed to take a closer look at our compatibility. I pray that this process will go quickly and they find the best match. Since we have to look nationwide, the process will take longer.

This delay means I will need to go through at least one consolidation round of chemo, if not two, to remain in remission. The consolidation chemo phase is very similar to what I went through in 2014-15. I will be in the hospital for six days and go home while my blood counts recover, getting lab work often to check for blood and platelet transfusions. I was very sad about this, but I understand it's necessary to make sure I stay in remission until we can move forward with the stem cell transplant. If none of these American donors are suitable for me, we will need to search worldwide. The waiting is the most challenging part. Not being able to speed up the process makes me feel powerless.

I have many appointments scheduled for labs over the next few weeks, which may also include blood and platelet transfusions. On June 22, I have an appointment with my doctor. During this visit, I hope to find out more about my donor and see when I need to return to the hospital for the consolidation chemo. I am not looking forward to more chemo, but this brings me another step closer to life.

 Joshua 1:9 ~ Have I not commanded you? Be strong and courageous. Do not be frightened, and do not be dismayed, for the Lord your God is with you.

A TWIST OF FATE

I was raised to believe that God has a plan for everyone and that seemingly random twists of fate are all a part of His plan.

~ Ronald Reagan

This week has been full of many trips to Nebraska Medicine for labs and blood transfusions. The past few days have been tough because I've felt terrible from body aches and a lingering low-grade fever. Tim tried to cheer me up by taking me for a drive to get out of the house, but I really didn't feel well and just wanted to do nothing. I had a strong feeling that my bone marrow was finally beginning to produce blood cells and platelets on its own. Believe me, I was so grateful for the regeneration, but this reboot is a painful process. Everyone knows that it's no fun to feel miserable. In times of struggle, I remind myself that tomorrow is another day closer to the goal.

On June 16, Tim came with me to the Fred & Pamela Buffett Cancer Center for a day of appointments. We met with my case manager, and she told me that they were still waiting for blood samples from the nationwide pool. Then she handed me a book with lots of information about graft-versus-host disease and the potential after-effects of stem cell transplants. She said reading it can be overwhelming at times, but I should just put it down when needed. This transplant sounds so scary, and the complications even scarier, but people make it through. I intend to overcome the odds as well – God willing.

My case manager also indicated that it's taking longer for my blood counts to rise on their own, so she wanted me to be prepared if the bone marrow biopsy scheduled for this afternoon showed that I'm not in remission. If that's the case, my chemo cocktail would need to be prepared for another long seven-day round. I told her that I refused to think anything other than remission. My body generally takes a while to recover, but it always circles back to good health with the aid of time. This slow recovery was very similar to my experiences in 2014. All the medical care team has to do is give me more time. I just know I'm in remission! I feel it in my heart.

Our meeting ended with my case manager saying she would call with the results of labs when she received them. Shortly after we left, Tim got the call from my case manager, and she informed us that my body was working on its own now! Hearing this news gave me a big sigh of relief.

My next appointment involved an echocardiogram to ensure my heart was still strong. Then a pulmonary function test to check my lungs. And last was a bone marrow biopsy and aspiration. On our way, I was thrilled to run into my friends from the hospital who had come to visit their nineteen-year-old son. Since Tim and I were early for my next appointment, we decided to briefly visit about how their son was doing. While we were chatting with them, my doctor (whom I've only met one time at this point) was walking down the hall. Tim asked, "Isn't that your doctor?" I said, "Yes!" When my doctor got closer, I stopped him and said, "You may not remember me because we only met once, but my name is Mary Robinson. I just saw my case manager and am so excited to hear that my bone marrow is working on its own now! It takes my body a little longer to kick in, so don't give up on me!" He shook my hand with a smile and said he wouldn't give up. Then, he walked away. I was so happy to have had an opportunity to see him. God set all this up – even seeing our new friends!

It was time to get checked in for my bone marrow biopsy. The medical staff was running behind schedule, and we had to wait. Tim got a text from the friends we had just seen, and it said that they wanted to give me something. Shortly after that, the mother of the nineteen-year-old son came to the waiting area with a beautiful homemade hard-covered book. One day while in the hospital, I told her about my rainbow miracles and how God had shown me that He was with me. She said it resonated with her, and she wanted to give me her book of nature photos that she had taken on their land. She also added scriptures from the Bible. A double rainbow is on the front cover, adorned with another Bible verse from Genesis 9:13 – "I have placed my rainbow in the clouds. It is the sign of my covenant with you and with all the earth." God brought our families together to help us get through this!

After twenty minutes, I still hadn't been called back for the bone marrow biopsy. Suddenly, my case manager approached us and canceled the procedure altogether. She said my doctor saw that my body was finally producing blood on its own, and they didn't want a false-positive biopsy. Since my body is just now beginning to work independently, it may have shown cancer blasts in the bone marrow when that wasn't really the case. Thank God she came before the biopsy started. Another miracle on my journey.

The receptionist rescheduled the bone marrow biopsy for five days from now. Hopefully, my body will be ready by then. They also postponed my appointment with my doctor to give my body more recovery time. Things are finally looking up!

 Jeremiah 29:11-12 ~ "For I know the plans I have for you," declares the Lord, "plans to prosper you and not to harm you, plans to give you hope and a future. Then you will call on me and come and pray to me, and I will listen to you."

Expression of Praise

On June 22, I woke up feeling refreshed. The birds were singing outside my window, as they do every morning this time of year. I was warm and cozy in bed with Tim by my side. The house was quiet, and I had a strong feeling that it was going to be a good day. In fact, this is the best I've felt since my last chemo treatment!

I decided to drive to my parents' house for some hot tea and light-hearted conversation to celebrate another 'stress' getting checked off my list yesterday – I completed another bone marrow biopsy and aspiration. Of course, I was very nervous during the procedure because of last time's hiccup with the electric drill, but this appointment was with a much more experienced physician assistant. She had been performing bone marrow biopsies for over twenty-five years. She eased my nerves by extracting the bone manually with a hand-held tool that she twisted while applying pressure. Everything went smoothly, and she assured me that she would be my personal bone marrow physician from now on.

Fortunately, I didn't need to wait long to hear that the preliminary results of my bone marrow biopsy confirmed that I am still in remission. The final results will take a few more days, but I don't doubt that they will be the same. Praise be to God! I was also informed that I would be admitted into the hospital for another round of chemo on June 26. This chemo will be high-dose (HiDAC), the same type I received in the consolidation phase in 2014. HiDAC means I'm going to go through six intense rounds of chemo, all crammed into five days. I will be allowed to go home to recover on the sixth day and might need to follow up with more blood and platelet transfusions until my bone marrow kicks in. The medical care team and I also discussed the stem cell donor again. After further testing, they had found too many potential graft-versus-host complications from the nationwide pool of possible donors. As a result, they opened up to a worldwide search and discovered five more possible matches. I am getting increasingly anxious as time goes by... I thought the process would have gone a lot faster.

However, as ready as I am, I cannot lie and say that I am not scared of the stem cell transplant. Many people have told me how hard it can be to make it through the side effects of graft-versus-host disease. I pray that the stem cells of my donor and I merge together perfectly. I am also worried about the recovery period after the transplant is completed. A hundred days of isolation with four kids sounds a bit easier said than done. I just pray everyone stays healthy. My doctor said it's best to be in my natural environment with those I love when I leave the hospital. I continue to pray that God's mighty forces guide the medical staff.

 Psalm 27:1 ~ The LORD is my light and my salvation — whom shall I fear? The LORD is the stronghold of my life — of whom shall I be afraid?

COURAGEOUS HEART

The only courage that matters is the kind
that gets you from one moment to the next.

~ Mignon McLaughlin

I was so glad to have last weekend with my family before returning to the hospital for the week-long stay of consolidation chemo treatment. Even if it's just sitting and watching a movie or playing a board game, time with loved ones calms my anxious mind. I've learned that simplicity is peaceful. Having said all this, my family and I were also very productive over the past couple of days. Three of my children got haircuts, and Shaylee cut off ten inches of her hair to send to *Wigs For Kids*. I am so proud of her! She wanted her hair short anyway, so it turned out to be an easy way to help another child in need.

Of course, June 26 came too quickly. My parents, Brody, and I went to the Fred & Pamela Buffett Cancer Center for labs. Brody was first, and they took six more vials of blood. Yikes! He was such a trooper and said it didn't hurt too much. He said, "Anything for you, Mom." My lab appointment was after that, and they took eight vials from me! I'm not sure what all of it was for, but I'm assuming it was mostly to recheck Brody's and my compatibility. I guess he is still 'Plan B' if the worldwide match doesn't work out. 'Plan A' would be the most preferable, but I'm glad to have a backup so we can move forward no matter what.

After I got checked in and settled into my room, a social worker from Nebraska Medicine stopped by to visit with me about some tough, but important, news. I was informed that I needed to appoint Tim as the Power of Attorney for Healthcare in case I am ever in a critical position and can't make rational decisions. The form is simple to fill out, but I anxiously cried when I read it. A couple of the items were about life-sustaining treatment and choosing whether or not to stop nutrition and hydration if it was too harmful for my body at any given time. I also needed to fill out a form regarding a Living Will Declaration. It was almost like signing off on the fact that I could die. If there were ever a time that life support was needed and doctors felt there wasn't a chance of survival, Tim would need to follow my wishes. Being forced to make preparations for the possibility of death felt very counterproductive for maintaining a positive frame of mind. I solemnly took the forms so Tim and I could discuss my wishes. Even though I was troubled, I refused to let these technicalities get in the way of my survival. Instead of thinking about frightening scenarios, I am opting to keep my heart and mind focused on my family.

My case manager came to visit with me shortly after the social worker left to talk about my new potential donors. They have three blood samples so far (not including the additional blood from Brody) and should have some concrete results by the end of this week. It sounds like things are finally moving along. I hope they have everything lined up before another HiDAC chemo treatment regimen becomes necessary for continued remission. This process seems to be taking such a long time. Isn't that funny? All I want is more time, but I don't have much more to waste. It's scary when your life depends on someone else.

On Friday, June 30, it was time for me to quit stalling and face reality with the Power of Attorney for Healthcare and Living Will Declaration forms. My social worker connected me with a lawyer to complete the process, and Nebraska Medicine took care of this cost. I was very grateful for everyone's assistance.

As the day went on, I became nauseous and sluggish. I feel like these are physical representations of the mental strain I've been dealing with upon reentry into the hospital. Nonetheless, the nurse gave me extra nausea medicine to hopefully ease the discomfort. Unfortunately, it didn't help much. I decided to sleep the afternoon away, and the extra rest helped more than anything. Tomorrow, I will get to go home and be with my precious family! All the pain is worth it.

 Proverbs 18:10 ~ The name of the Lord is a strong tower; the righteous man runs into it and is safe.

HOPE BURNING BRIGHT

Friends are like flowers blooming in the spring.
They are beautiful and priceless, like a diamond ring.
They are like pearls, which are unique and rare.
They are loving and warm, like a teddy bear.
What I'm trying to say is that friends are the best.
And since I have one like this, I know I am blessed.

~ Holly Robinson, my daughter (written when she was young)

Since returning home from the hospital last Saturday, July 1, many things have happened – some of them not so good. My eyes went through a side effect that I would prefer never to happen again. Memories of this extremely painful occurrence came rushing back because the same thing happened to me in 2014. Even though the medical care team had prescribed steroid eye drops to help protect my eyes from the chemo's wrath, it still didn't seem to work. For nearly three days this week, every time I blinked, it felt like my eyeballs were being gouged out with fingernails. Natural light wasn't kind to my eyes either. I wore sunglasses everywhere, including in the house and during lab appointments. It was easiest for me to just rest on the couch with my eyes shut, hoping for the pain to subside on its own. It seemed like I tried everything to make it go away, including but not limited to moisturizing eye drops, ziplock baggies of cool water, slices of raw potato, tea bags, and a frozen eye gel pad. All of this effort with no luck.

Fortunately, Holly is taking excellent care of me until Tim's return home. I guess my eye pain just needs to run its course. On the evening of July 3, I received a group text from a couple of my close friends, inviting my family to shoot off fireworks with them. I was so excited for my children because they will still enjoy the Fourth of July this year. I would never want my health to stand in the way of events that only come once a year. My friends said they would take care of everything! They brought snacks and drinks, along with a variety of fireworks, to our family cabin. The expressions on my kids' faces were priceless. Everyone had a blast together. The help of my friends gave me so much relief.

I even got to join in on a bit of the fun from my seat inside the cabin. I watched the fireworks through the window the entire evening, and when anyone came in for snacks, I briefly visited with them. It was the best Fourth of July I could ask for. My eyes were feeling slightly better at that point, but I still needed to wear sunglasses because bright lights proceeded to bother them. Even so, it brought back memories of the carefree lighting of fireworks as a child. Fireworks have always inspired feelings of freedom; they seem to transmit the illusion that all is well in the world. And just as the lights burst and leave behind memories of valor and strength, I have hope that my CANcer will leave a bright mark upon completion. My sickness has a purpose, and its final image is significant, even with all the ugliness in-between.

The entire evening was perfect, and I thanked God for the support of my friends. They made the night so special for my family. Friends always seem to know what we need, even when we don't ask. Sometimes we forget the value of relationships. I especially appreciate their assistance now that I'm in such desperate need, but I've come to realize the importance of recognizing the little things too. A small favor can go a long way.

 1 Thessalonians 5:11 ~ Therefore encourage one another and build each other up, just as in fact you are doing.

Realistically Idealistic

While waiting for my lab results on July 17, I decided to begin reading the graft-versus-host disease book that my case manager gave me a month ago. I had been putting it off because I knew the complications would be overwhelming. I got to page seventeen and had to put it down. The book began with chronic conditions that could happen to some individuals with allogeneic (donor) stem cell transplants (the kind I'm having). My paranoia intensified with each sentence I read and each page I turned. I thought to myself, "Why do they give this dreadful book to all of us awaiting a stem cell transplant?" I was doing well, staying mentally strong and holding it all together until the potential tortures of my future were laid out for me. Knowledge is not always power. I realize I need to be aware of possible problems, but this black and white information is not helping me in my current state.

I was very emotional, weeping off and on for the next couple of days. Tim was out of town again for the week, so I relied on my mom to keep my spirits intact. She hung out with the kids and me for most of the day and kept me busy with projects that were on my 'to-do' list.

I visited with my case manager over the phone on July 18. She told me that I needed to schedule labs, an educational meeting, and a visit with my doctor on July 27. She said he might want to give me another round of chemo called Vidaza before the stem cell transplant to ensure I remain in remission. Vidaza, apparently, was a five-day chemo regimen that lasted approximately an hour each day. It's an outpatient treatment, and most people tolerate it well. Of course, I hope that I don't have to do it, but it doesn't sound too horrible, so I will follow whatever their protocol recommends.

Since I had my case manager on the phone, I told her that I preferred to hold off on reading the graft-versus-host book she gave me. In fact, I didn't even have access to the book at that point. A friend (an angel) saw how upset I was and took it from me. She said she would read it for me so I didn't have to and promised that she would return it when the time was right. I felt relieved that the book was out of my hands. Maybe I'll finish reading it later, or at least look into parts of it (as my case manager suggested during our conversation), but for now, I'm going to rely on my body to tell me if something is not quite feeling right. I can contact my medical care team from there. Theoretical issues swarming around in my mind are only hindering the completion of this final stretch.

I also asked my case manager if there was another option instead of the stem cell transplant because, at that point, I was second-guessing if the risks were worth it. She said that if I didn't follow through with the procedure, I would need to continue chemo regimens for the rest of my life. Chemo can only go so far, and, eventually, it wouldn't be enough to keep me alive. The transplant is my best option for a cure. If that's what it takes, so be it.

I received another book about allogeneic stem cell transplants from my case manager in the mail a few days later. It looks like a much lighter read. I am doing my best to move forward confidently. Fortunately, I have the help of my herbalist. He is preparing me emotionally and physically for the stem cell transplant through natural tinctures, effectively eliminating foreign invaders with herbs. And yes, my oncologist has known about this extra medicine and continues to be supportive. The only time I'm not allowed to take oral herbs is during chemo treatments and hospital stays. However, even with that limitation, I'm still allowed to use some essential oils topically while in the hospital. Our compromise has been serving me well.

There is a weekly support group at the Fred & Pamela Buffett Cancer Center for leukemia and lymphoma patients awaiting a stem cell transplant or who have had one in the past. They meet over the lunch hour and provide a nice meal for us to eat while we chat. I have wanted to go ever since my social worker told me about it, and I figured this was the perfect week to do it. I asked my mom if she would go with me, and, of course, since there was food involved, she eagerly agreed. Shaylee even asked if she could join too!

My mom, Shaylee, and I felt immediately welcomed when we arrived at the meeting. My social worker is in charge of the group, and her energy is so helpful and supportive. Everyone introduced themselves, and the discussion began. It was very informal, and anyone could speak about whatever was on their mind. Occasionally, my social worker would facilitate discussions to focus on specific topics. I was the only one in attendance who had not had a stem cell transplant yet. It was reassuring for me to actually 'see' and visit with those who have been through it. One individual was a little over thirty days out, another was over one hundred days, and some a year or more out. They spoke about their experiences, and their positive stories eased my mind. I was so glad to have gone.

Tim came with me to the weekly support meeting the following week to pass the time before my scheduled appointments. Again, the conversations were delightful. There were familiar faces and some new ones. Tim and I plan to attend as often as possible. A friend who also participated in the meeting said that someone told her, "Everyone who has gone through cancer has been touched by God." Her philosophy is so true. CANcer is just another large mountain to climb, and I know I'm equipped with all the spiritual gear necessary to make it to the top. One of my favorite sayings is, "If God brings you to it, He will bring you through it!"

After the meeting, we dashed to my appointment with the lawyer to sign documents for my 'Last Will and Testament.' God willing, we won't need to worry about this for many years, but it's critical to be prepared. I asked Tim to put the finalized forms in our safe at home to help me erase the written plans from my mind. I'm not going to die just yet.

Following the lawyer's session, Tim and I went to an educational meeting with my case manager. While there, we received a 'blue book,' as she called it. It held everything I needed to know about my upcoming chemo regimen, including the steps leading to the stem cell transplant and possible side effects. Similar to the book about graft-versus-host disease, this blue book brought me close to tears. I learned awful things, like how my toenails and fingernails could fall off! I hate having to understand the not-so-pretty side of recovery.

When my case manager had finished introducing me to the cursed book, I had an appointment with my doctor. He told me that my blood work looked good. We discussed many things, and he mentioned that I should do well with the transplant. They use a program that gives patients a survival score based on all test results – with zero being the best score. I have a score of two, which is considered very good. Some patients have much higher scores. My score is two because of the results from my pulmonary test. I told him that my lungs were getting better every day because I was doing what he recommended – daily exercise until the transplant date to keep up my strength and help me get through it. Generally, people lose ten to twenty pounds after receiving transplants.

We also discussed Vidaza chemo and whether or not he feels I need an additional round since the transplant is only one week later than initially planned. I was so relieved when he said, "One week really doesn't make a difference in your case." He told me to enjoy the time I had before the procedure. Tim asked if we could celebrate and eat dinner at a restaurant since my blood counts were up. And, once again, I was thrilled when my doctor approved it! I still need to be cautious, but it's comforting to know that I can spend some time outdoors, hug my friends, and cuddle with my kids. God is so good!

 Philippians 4:6 ~ Do not be anxious about anything, but in every situation, by prayer and petition, with thanksgiving, present your requests to God.

THE MAGIC OF NUMBERS

The universe is always speaking to us. Sending us little messages,
causing coincidences and serendipities, reminding us to stop,
to look around, to believe in something else, something more.

~ Nancy Thayer

It's already July 28. Time is moving quickly, and I'm starting to wonder if I'll ever find a suitable donor. But, by the grace of God, I finally received a phone call from my case manager this morning. She said that since they had no luck finding a donor nationwide, they searched worldwide and found three, ten-out-of-ten matches. Interestingly enough, they were ALL forty-eight years old – one female and two males.

My doctor preferred males, so we eliminated the female from the mix before further testing. One male is blood type A positive, and the other is blood type B. My blood type is O Positive, the universal donor, but I'm not quite sure about how relevant that is to the transplant's compatibility. After the stem cell transplant, my blood type will gradually shift to the donor's type. His stem cells will marry into my body, and we will become one.

After several meetings with the medical care team and a closer analysis of both donors' DNA, my doctor chose the male with the A positive blood for my match. I smiled and said, "It fits me well – A positive," and the number **48** also resonated with me – 4+8 is **12**, which is a master number, a number of God, and one that carries a divine message. Twelve is a symbol of faith and purpose, a number to inspire one to take action. It represents the presence of Angels. It is also said to signify positivity, faithfulness, optimism, and growth.

The **number 12** is featured prominently in the **Bible**. The Old Testament Book of Genesis states there were **12** sons of Jacob, and those **12** sons formed the **12** tribes of Israel. The New Testament tells us that Jesus had **12** disciples. With the donor found and confirmed, we scheduled August 15 for the stem cell transplant. And here's where **12** gets even more interesting and where my faith gave me a gentle nod that everything would work out in the best way possible for me at this time. My donor had prior obligations on the pre-scheduled date of August 15 for the stem cell transplant. The week after worked better for him, so the new date was set for August 22, the day I was baptized as an infant. Since August is the eighth month, and the big day is the twenty-second, 8+2+2 also adds up to **12**. As a final thought, my birthday is August 2; 8+2 is **10. Number 10** represents rebirth, assertiveness, and professional leadership. It's also the number of new beginnings.

God has this in the palm of His hand. His ways are ingenious, and methods are sure. Blessings of peace arose within me. In my heart, I knew this final stage for long-term wellness would have a positive outcome. I just needed to let my heart lead the way and prevent fearful thoughts from taking over. God has the perfect plan for me – for all of us. I will trust in Him always.

My stem cell transplant date is one week later than initially planned. Now I might need another week-long round of chemo (consolidation phase) before I'm admitted into the hospital for the transplant. I will be hospitalized for this extra round of chemo for about six days. Initially, my heart sank a bit. I was not looking forward to more treatments.

I came to the conclusion that even though the stem cell transplant was pushed back a week, it was a good sign to have the transplant on the day I was baptized. This procedure will be like another rebirth, and I will have two birthdays for the rest of my life. My case manager said, "Even though your 'real' birthday is August 2, your family needs to make sure they celebrate your second birthday on August 22, too! It's a very important date to remember." I can handle that! Who doesn't like to celebrate and eat yummy desserts? I know this girl does! Come to think of it, why not go all-in? An entire month of birthday celebrations sounds more like it! I can picture it now: Queen Mary will have her family wait on her every desire. After all, I've earned it.

 Jeremiah 29:11 ~ "For I know the plans I have for you," declares the Lord, "plans to prosper you and not to harm you, plans to give you hope and a future."

THE FUTURE UNFOLDING
ONE STEP AT A TIME

We must let go of the life we had planned,
so as to accept the life that is waiting for us.

~ Joseph Cambell

Do you ever wonder what the future holds? What would be different if you chose to proceed left instead of right? How would the consequences of this decision shape your life and those you love? Would it open doors for new experiences? Alternatively, would it erase opportunities that would have popped up from continuing straight ahead?

Only God knows the answers to these questions, and His Spiritual Team guides us in the most appropriate direction. However, even with their divine guidance, it's up to us to choose whether we want to follow our destined routes or not. Sometimes thorns and branches block our path, or a thick fog forces us to turn around. Other times, the road is perfectly clear. Pray for this clarity, meditate on your future, and wait for the fog to lift. Trust that God is by your side.

I've thought about the future a lot lately. I'm not sure what my life is going to look like after the stem cell transplant. Will I have the stamina to accomplish the hefty goals that my former self took so seriously? To be honest, there's not much I can do about that right now aside from wait. So, in the meantime, I breathe in comfort – breathe out worry, breathe in courage and confidence – breathe out fear. Inhaling goodness (peace, forgiveness, love, joy, etc.) and exhaling toxins (anger, stress, bitterness, guilt, etc.) provides relief like nothing else. And it works for less-serious stressors too! Sometimes we all just need to take a big breath when we're overwhelmed with parenthood, job difficulties, or annoying tasks. Humans are capable of so much, and we can get through anything when we establish a proper frame of mind.

A few nights ago, I was in bed quieting my thoughts with routine prayer and deep-breathing exercises. This time, I also decided to ask God what I needed to work on. I expected something like patience with the kids or remaining even-tempered when my house isn't in order, but He replied with something completely different. I heard God tell me, "Passion." He said I need to figure out what sets fire to my soul, lights up my life, and makes me whole. It was a reminder not to let my attention wander. Imagine what will happen if I focus on my passions. I will finally grow into the person He has destined for me to become.

Have you given thought to what lights you up and adds zest to your life? If you still haven't figured out your drive, quiet your mind and ask God to help you. Feel His presence surround you, opening doors that lead to happiness and health. If you feel moved to do so, take a leap of faith. If you're waiting for permission, give it to yourself. You are worthy of greatness.

On another note, I have been feeling great these past couple of weeks. On July 31, my bone marrow biopsy and labs went well. I was ecstatic when my case manager wrote me an email with the final results and this statement: "Your bone marrow biopsy was fabulously NORMAL. Not a genetic mark, etcetera… Beautiful." That was the best news ever and a much-awaited response to my prayer request! I also learned that I would not need another consolidation chemo treatment before the stem cell transplant.

As the transplant date drew closer, I became more apprehensive. I decided to go back for another support group meeting to boost my spirits. It eased my mind to be with people who understood how I felt. A gentleman I hadn't seen before came to the Leukemia and Lymphoma support group on August 4. He mentioned that he didn't come very often, but I sure got a kick out of his spunky personality and felt he went to this meeting for a reason – to ease my nerves about death. It happened to be his four-year anniversary (post-transplant), and he looked great!

He had the most remarkable story! In his late sixties, this man had a cardiopulmonary arrest (heart stopped beating) several months after his stem cell transplant due to graft-versus-host disease. He told the group that he waited too long to call the doctor about his symptoms, which included extreme diarrhea and fatigue. By the time he sought help, it was almost too late. The ambulance was taking him to the hospital when he coded, and the paramedics vigilantly worked to revive him. During this time, he had a vision: A short distance from him was a sparkling waterfall plummeting down from a high point, surrounded by fog, or possibly the mist of the water toppling into the pool beneath. Slowly, his loved ones came into sight from the misty vapor. They cheerfully walked toward him – his dad was first, mom was second (she was the most animated of the bunch, waving her arm and motioning him to come to them), and last was a relative holding his infant son, who had passed away at twenty-one days old.

They all had smiles and were delighted to see him. While all this was happening, he was like a statue and couldn't move. After some time (he doesn't recall how long), they all began to walk back into the misty vapor and could no longer be seen. Then he opened his eyes, and the paramedic said, "I think we have him back." The paramedic told him that it took about fifteen minutes to revive him. He was so grateful to see his loved ones on the other side and knew they would be reunited when it was his time to go. He was not done with his life yet.

This story is so encouraging! I needed to hear it since I might also be on the brink of death with my upcoming stem cell transplant. There is no doubt in my mind that heaven exists. It might look different for each of us, but hearing this man's story took some of the fear away. When it's my time to go, I will be just fine, in a serene dwelling surrounded by love. That doesn't matter right now, though, for I have this deep sense that my time on Earth is not finished yet.

And just to reaffirm that I will make it through this trial, God gave me a sign from my daughter Shaylee. Recently, Colby and Shaylee were away with some family friends for a much-needed fun-filled week of just being kids. When they returned, Shaylee gave me two gifts; the first was a canvas painted with a beautiful tree that she finished herself, and the second was a rock with the words "Have Faith" engraved in it. These unexpected treasures were just what I needed to lift my spirits. I adore both presents and will take them to the hospital with me, placing them beside the other items that give me comfort.

Shaylee went with me to the Fred & Pamela Buffett Cancer Center on Thursday, August 10, for a long day of appointments and attended the support group meeting with me. At the end of each session, a container filled with candy is handed around the table. Each person has the opportunity to share some words of wisdom and grab a sweet treat when the container is passed to them. When it was Shaylee's turn to trade off advice, she said, "If you woke up this morning, God's not through with you yet." Amen to that! I was so proud of her for speaking in front of a large group and for understanding something with such deep truth. It's even more profound that she meaningfully participated in a giving-and-receiving exercise. It makes me happy to know that my children are also learning from my bout of illness. This CANcer has a purpose.

 Proverbs 3:16-18 ~ Long life is in her right hand; in her left hand are riches and honor. Her ways are pleasant ways, and all her paths are peace. She is a tree of life to those who take hold of her; those who hold her fast will be blessed.

CELLS BRING BACK LIFE

I have learned, as a rule of thumb, never to ask whether you can do something. Say, instead, that you are doing it. Then fasten your seatbelt. The most remarkable things follow.

~ Julia Cameron

There is a chapter about health in the book *The Secret* by Rhonda Bryne. It states that "healing through the mind can work harmoniously with medicine" and that we need to "think perfect health" no matter what is happening around us. I'm finding mindfulness to be so necessary, and I will continue to manifest my perfect health through purposeful prayer, meditation, and healing energy.

Tuesday, August 15, seemed to arrive quickly. Tim drove me to the hospital to start the intense chemo treatments on 'day negative six,' preparing for 'day zero' of the transplant. Unwanted nerves came rushing back when I was admitted back into the hospital. The stem cell transplant was real, and it was finally happening. Even though the cursed images from my case manager's blue book started creeping back into my mind, I continued my pursuit of good health with positivity and walked confidently to my room.

My doctor said to expect three to four additional weeks in the hospital after the procedure was completed. During this stay, I would be given specific medications to counter any potential complications that may show up. One drug, in particular, focused wholly on the prevention of graft-versus-host disease. It was also my job to help the doctors watch for signs of the disease, ensuring that they could stop the cell rejection as soon as possible. If any reactions get too out of control, my body will start attacking itself until death. Let's hope my match and I are perfectly compatible! The supreme team!

Tim helped me settle into my new room, and the final chemo regimen began. Until this point, I knew exactly what to expect from my treatments because I went through the same protocol in 2014. This unfamiliar phase is frightening. Hopefully, this initial discomfort is for nothing, and my body will react seamlessly to these foreign chemo cocktails. I continued to pray for only my highest good to ease my nerves. This regimen called for five days of intense chemotherapy, followed by my stem cell transplant. Sounds simple enough.

It's easier said than done, though, because I began suffering from intense nausea and vomiting after only three days of chemo. The medical care team did what they could to quickly settle my stomach during these episodes, but it didn't get much better. I slept a lot and pushed through seemingly-endless bouts of fevers, chills, body aches, and rashes. Even though I was asleep most of the time, Tim and my children stopped by often and always helped lift my spirits. It's just nice to know that my loved ones are here to care for me.

Routine has been essential in keeping me moving, so I always try my best to keep a daily schedule: Eat small bits of food, shower, and walk the hallway. I even went to the outdoor Healing Garden as often as possible to get fresh air and be in nature, even if I wasn't always in the mood to do so. Bumblebees and butterflies made multiple appearances and fluttered about the beautiful plant life and flowers. Peaceful music was always playing softly from speakers speckled throughout the area. Sometimes a breeze would dance on my skin and provide a temporary sense of security and comfort. The reassurance that the world was still out there was just what I needed to muster up the strength to move forward.

On Sunday, August 20, Tim called to tell me the title of the Pastor's sermon: 'God Rewards Perseverance.' Impeccable timing, if you ask me. I will continue to show perseverance, and I genuinely feel that my ambition will be rewarded with a long and fruitful life. God has abundant plans for me.

Ephesians 3:20-21 ~ Now to him who is able to do immeasurably more than all we ask or imagine, according to his power that is at work within us, to him be glory in the church and in Christ Jesus throughout all generations, for ever and ever! Amen.

The DNA of a LEO Lion

I was so sick during the transplant preparation period that I didn't take much time to journal. It's finally day zero, August 22, and my stem cell transplant is complete. Now I only need four more doses of chemo to finalize the process. It's pretty common for patients in this stage to complain of terrible sore throats – just another chemotherapy side effect – and I pray that I'm one of the few who remain unaffected. I've heard it's incredibly unpleasant. The last few days have had a few ups and a lot of downs, but I know it will all be over soon. I can't wait until this last step is behind me and I get to go home. With all that being said, the main message to take from all this is that I've been reborn!

 Matthew 11:28-30 ~ "Come to me, all you who are weary and burdened, and I will give you rest. Take my yoke upon you and learn from me, for I am gentle and humble in heart, and you will find rest for your souls. For my yoke is easy and my burden is light. "

WE CAN'T BE POSITIVE ALL THE TIME

Sometimes the strength within you is not a big fiery flame
for all to see, it is just a tiny spark that whispers
ever so softly, "You got this. Keep going."

~ Unknown

My courage is under fire! It's now twelve days after the stem cell transplant, and I find each day to be a struggle. Currently, I have a feeding tube because my throat hurts too terribly to eat solid food or take oral medication. The sore throat is a side effect of Methotrexate chemotherapy. Fortunately, I only have one more dose that my nurse will give me today. The chemo literally melts a layer of skin off my throat, burning all the way down through my digestive tract and causing mouth sores in the process. My doctor said that once my white blood count begins to rise on its own, my throat will heal quickly. I'm still nauseous and experiencing occasional vomiting, but the medical care team is slowly getting my symptoms under control. Blood and platelet transfusions are proving to be a must for survival. Lord, please help me remain strong through this phase.

I feel so weak and am having difficulty standing on solid ground. I find myself slipping in and out of my perceived positive mindset. Do I genuinely think I can get through this? Is it even possible? Negativity is probably a normal reaction, but I'm just so surprised by how unprepared I was for this extent of pain. I'm not sure if I truly knew what I signed up for. Enduring the transplant's effects happens to be the most difficult process I've ever been through in my entire life. I wish I had a fast-forward button.

I lie on my hospital bed with tears streaming down my cheeks and glance out the window, hoping to capture some brief evidence of nature. The sky is blue and empty. I wish there was more life. Shifting my sight to the decorated wall across from my bed, I observe our collage of family photos. Cherished memories seep back, and I begin to remember what I'm fighting for in the first place. A smile creeps in through my tears of misery, and I force myself back into the light.

Taking a deep breath, I wipe the tears and remind myself that God IS with me. My family is cheering me on, and I AM willing to do what it takes to make it out of the torture device doctors like to call 'stem cell transplants.' I visualize myself as healthy and drift off to sleep with the nearly-forgotten comfort of positivity.

 Isaiah 41:10 ~ So do not fear, for I am with you; do not be dismayed, for I am your God. I will strengthen you and help you; I will uphold you with my righteous right hand.

I CALLED FOR COURAGE, AND TIM'S MESSAGE BOLSTERS ME

No relationship is all sunshine, but two people can share one umbrella and survive the storm together.

~ Anonymous

"To my beautiful wife, Mary Jane Robinson. I cannot put into words how proud I am of you. The Lord certainly broke the mold when he made you. I am a very lucky man to be the husband of such a gorgeous, loving, giving, spiritual, and passionate woman. The sky's the limit with Mary!

You are the best thing that has ever touched my life, and you have made me the man I am today. You are an unbelievably loving mother of our four incredible children, who are all very unique, each in their own way. You overflow with goodness that anyone who's ever had the privilege of being in your presence can feel. You have an inner strength that is unmatched by any man or woman I've ever met, and I want you to know that the kids and I are so proud of your perseverance.

You are fighting the battle of your life. This extremely difficult challenge is one that most would not have the strength to overcome. There is no doubt in my heart that you are not only going to keep fighting, but you are going to come out victorious because you wield the secret weapon: GOD. I know that our Lord has something special planned for your future. I'm not exactly sure what it is yet, but I know it will have something to do with your compassion to help others. Empathy is one of your very best traits. It is something that God has put directly into your heart since birth. Whatever God has planned for the future, there is no doubt in my mind that it will be spectacular – just like you.

I know there's still a tough road ahead, but know that you (WE) are up for the challenge! We will see this trial through by the grace of God. I am so excited to see what He has in store for our family! You have always been a fighter, and I know that you will win this one. You can give CANcer another kick in the ass for me while you have it pinned down!

We all miss you so much. Our home has been incomplete without you in it. Hurry up and get better so you can come home where you belong! I love you with my whole heart, always and forever!

Your Loving Husband, Tim"

 Proverbs 16:24 ~ Gracious words are a honeycomb, sweet to the soul and healing to the bones.

What a Difference a Few Days Makes

It's September 6, and I received a unit of blood because my hemoglobin was low, but my platelets are over two hundred! Praise be to God for my continued recovery. He is my rock, strength, and refuge. I will never grow weary with Him by my side.

Today is also the day that I got my feeding tube out! I may or may not have caused a scene with my nurse, ordering her to remove it from my nose, but no matter the tactics, I got the job done! It was worth it, too, because I felt like the tube was starting to make me gag and choke on my spit. My throat was killing me, and that seemed to be the only way to get some relief.

I'm also thrilled to hear that I'll be discharged from the hospital sometime later today. I told my doctor that "home is where you heal." He agreed and decided to let me go home a few days early. I've been stuck in the hospital for over three weeks now. My mouth sores and throat still hurt immensely, but my doctor trusts I will be able to drink enough fluids during my home recovery, despite the pain. My blood levels will recover faster if I stay hydrated, so I will do my best to drink more frequently. All I need to do now is remain focused, and my body should take care of the rest on its own. My outlook on life is positive from here on out. Before Tim and I head home, the nurses insist on giving me a unit of electrolytes to help with hydration.

Once I go home, I will still need to return to the hospital for several appointments, lab work, and PICC dressing changes. I need to call if there are any suspicions regarding graft-versus-host disease, fevers, chills, or other concerning symptoms. My doctor will monitor and update my medications twice a week, keeping a close eye on my needs. It's a downhill slope from here.

1 Peter 5:7 ~ Cast all your anxiety on him because he cares for you.

It's Not Easy, But It Is Worth It

It's now September 16. Sitting on the couch seems like my new routine these days. I often find myself looking at the piano that Holly plays so gracefully, practicing for her upcoming lessons. An assortment of photos of the kids adorns the top ledge of the piano, and in the middle of all those photos is a picture of Jesus, nicely framed with the words, "I never said it would be easy. I only said it would be worth it." It was given to me by a church member in 2014 when I was going through early rounds of treatments. For me, this is a constant yet gentle reminder that good days are yet to come, and God has been with me every step of the way.

This last stage of healing has been the most difficult one to go through, by far. It has been a terrifying and bumpy roller coaster of a ride, and every day I am reminded of how precious life is, along with what lengths I am willing to go to survive. I want nothing more than to be here with my family for many years. I don't want to miss out on anything – activities with the kids, graduations, marriages, becoming a grandmother... the list goes on and on. I have faith that this stem cell transplant will give me the precious time I yearn for.

Not to be a "Debbie Downer," but I need to make this real. I had sores that went from my mouth all the way down to my anus. It was not a fun ride. I needed to use a saliva ejector – a straw-like suction tube – to remove saliva from my mouth because it hurt so badly to swallow, and I choked annoyingly often, sometimes throwing up while trying to breathe. The feeding tube was an immense help when I couldn't eat or take my medicine due to throat pain, even though I hated using it.

As of today, my sore throat is almost healed, and I am so thankful. It felt like a fireball exploded every time I went to the bathroom, as if diarrhea wasn't enough on its own. Nausea and vomiting were my constant daily companions. My groin area turned dark purple from burnt, peeling skin, not to mention the terrible itch associated with it, which aggravated the site even more. These were all side effects of the intense chemo and transplant regimen. I tried to alleviate the pain with as many natural remedies as I could think of, but nothing was much help. I took baths with essential oils and Epsom salt, smeared aloe vera all over my body, and applied cool compresses on my burnt skin.

I pray that my quality of life improves so that I can fully enjoy the freedom that remission will provide. Right now, the dreary days seem to last forever, and I'm looking for any sign of relief from the pain. Perhaps things will start looking up tomorrow.

 Deuteronomy 31:6 ~ Be strong and courageous. Do not be afraid or terrified because of them, for the Lord your God goes with you; he will never leave you nor forsake you.

Healing Daily

As I continue to recover, I've noted that my mouth sores have disappeared entirely, my throat is almost healed, I haven't thrown up in four days, and it doesn't burn when I go to the bathroom anymore (although I still have loose stools). The skin on my groin, hands, arms, neck, armpits, and heels still bothers me, but I have been applying a prescribed steroid cream to soothe them. My hands and heels were the most blistered – it felt like they had been stuck on kabobs and roasted over a fire. The steroid cream has helped a bit, and the dead skin is beginning to peel.

All of my fingernails and a couple of toenails also felt the wrath of chemo. Each of them broke away from my cuticle and slowly fell off. My doctor indicated that the rashes on my arms were most likely due to graft-versus-host disease, but only a biopsy could determine his theory for sure. My emotional state of mind isn't ready for a biopsy yet. I have been poked and prodded enough. So, I've decided to wait and see what my doctor says at my appointment next week.

Since being released from the hospital, I have been going to the doctor twice a week. In the morning, I go in for lab work at one location, and in the afternoon, I see a healthcare provider at another. I hear that I am doing remarkably well at this point, and they are very pleased with my progress. Some people are still in the hospital at this stage or are using a wheelchair to get to appointments. I am very grateful for my steady recovery, but I still find myself in tears at times. I just wish I felt better and had more energy. I know this will all become a distant memory one day. I must push on.

The pain and fear are real, but I pray my hope permeates the darkness and is enough to cure this illness. Thank goodness I have an army of supporters lifting me in prayer! My daily mantra: "All is well," is with me at each turn. With this mantra, I also keep my children in my thoughts. I will be here to see them blossom and grow. Graft-versus-host disease is no match for my faith, courage, and tenacity.

 Jeremiah 17:14 ~ Heal me, LORD, and I will be healed; save me and I will be saved, for you are the one I praise.

Lean on Jesus

When I was a young child, I recall a framed poem on the wall in my parents' bedroom titled, *Footprints In The Sand* by Margaret Fishback Powers. It always had a way of generating spiritual goosebumps on my body when I read the last few lines stating: "He whispered, 'My precious child, I love you and will never leave you, never, ever, during your trials and testings. When you saw only one set of footprints, it was then that I carried you.'"

As I came up to the most challenging point in my life, I remembered this poem by Margaret Fishback Powers and learned that my Lord did indeed carry me when I didn't have the strength to do so on my own. It is because of Him that I see both sets of footprints in the sand again. Whenever doubts corrupted my mind, I returned to this poem and visualized the Lord and me walking side-by-side in the sand, admiring a brilliant shoreline together. When I became faint, unable to muster up enough strength to take any more steps, He said, "Take heart, dear child," and swept me off my feet. As I rested my weary head on His mighty shoulder and he cradled me with the most divine healing power, Jesus whispered, "Tomorrow, the sun will rise again and begin a new day. Rest now. Your faith has restored you."

 Psalm 121:1-2 ~ I lift up my eyes to the mountains — where does my help come from? My help comes from the Lord, the Maker of heaven and earth.

SEVEN

THE RIGHT AMOUNT OF THUNDER AND LIGHTNING

It's nearly impossible to achieve goals without temporarily sacrificing comfort. Risks and leaps of faith may feel unsafe or illogical in the moment, but sometimes they're the only way we can make progress. In more recent years, I have learned that risks help overcome fears of rejection, betrayal, failure, and even guilt. Some of the forgotten friendships of my past would have dissolved if I hadn't dared to reach out. Ultimately, stepping out of our safety bubble is essential when it comes to understanding the way of the world. Of course, sometimes curiosity leads us to places we're not supposed to go, but how would we learn not to stick our hand on the stove if we didn't feel the burn? Perhaps wounds fester into transformations, improving both our outlook and our abilities. What is success without a bit of underlying pain?

Nowadays, I refuse to hide behind dark curtains with my guard up at all times – life is way too short to let the 'what ifs' hold you back from great adventures. Plus, if you don't somehow release your negative feelings, they have the potential to morph into physical calamities, like, in my case, an illness. Embrace all experiences, no matter the emotion they may trigger. Think about how the low points of your life have helped define the person you have become.

SERVING SIZE MATTERS

Take little bites of bravery.

~ Lady Gaga

It's September 26, and I'm amazed at what a difference just a few days can make on one's health and attitude. Last week, I found myself teetering on the edge of an emotional mudslide. It took all I had to trudge through the thick sludge and maintain my mental balance. Thankfully, God heard all the prayers that were sent my way and saved me from this gloomy descent. I hear my army of supporters telling me to "Hang in there – it will get better." However, sometimes I wonder, "Will it get better? How does anyone know?" I suppose my faith-led journey is proof enough as I continue with each breath and positive step toward wellness. However, as I look to the Bible for comfort, I read, "Be still before the Lord and wait patiently for him." (Psalm 37:7) And sometimes, that's what we need to do for answers. Here's a recap of what happened:

On Tuesday, September 19, my doctor confirmed that I not only had side effects from the chemo (burnt skin, itchy, blisters, rashes), but I also had a mild case of graft-versus-host disease. Although I was initially devastated by this news, my doctor mentioned that graft-versus-host is not necessarily a terrible thing. We want a small amount of push-back because this means the stem cell transplant worked!

Currently, I am on a high dose of Prednisone to help alleviate symptoms. They will taper me off it when the time is right. My skin still itches (everywhere), and I still have a couple of blisters that have popped and are peeling in various locations, but I feel so much better. The most significant development is that I no longer have a terrible sore throat. Food is tasting better every day, and I'm gaining back weight!

On Sunday, I was ecstatic that my body was letting me eat, and the meal actually tasted good! Holly and I prepared a fresh pot of ham and potato soup. We added celery, carrots, cabbage, and onions to the broth. In my mind, I was so proud of myself for eating healthy. Unfortunately, I overindulged because it was just so yummy! Plus, it felt so good to actually be able to keep down food.

Unfortunately, the soup had a not-so-enjoyable side effect. I had to get up three times in the middle of the night to go to the bathroom, then another two times in the morning – all diarrhea. I decided to call my case manager and check if it was from the extra magnesium I had been taking. Sadly, that's not the news I heard at all. She told me to come to the hospital as soon as possible and pack a bag just in case they chose to admit me. My heart sank, and I instantly became terrified. She said it could be graft-versus-host disease in the stomach or bowels, and they may need to do further testing.

Since Tim was working out of town, my parents have been taking care of the kids and me by transporting us to appointments and school. So, my dad came to my house and drove me to Fred & Pamela Buffett Cancer Center that morning. I tried my best not to worry about what was to come.

Shortly after our arrival, a physician assistant came in and talked to me about the next steps. He drew some blood and mentioned that a stool sample would be helpful. The physician assistant said that I was going to be admitted into the hospital with no food or drink, just IV fluids, and the plan was to sedate me for a stomach and bowel biopsy the following day. It took only seconds for my complete freak-out to start.

I began to cry harder than I ever have before, sputtering out reasons why I needed to go home instead. I was in a crazed panic and had to force myself to take deep breaths. Honestly, I felt better than I had in weeks, and my rashes were improving tremendously. There was no reason for me to go back to the hospital, and all those additional tests sounded like they would just make me feel worse. I couldn't fathom why we needed to have such an extreme reaction so quickly. No matter what I think, however, I'm not the one in charge.

Through tears, I asked my dad to bring my suitcase from the truck and told him that he was going home without me. I continued with my emotional rampage as I sat in the room alone, waiting for my next orders, when my doctor suddenly stepped into my room. It was a miracle that he had come to see me! I wondered if someone had called him because I was so upset. I'm sure the other patients and staff could hear my episode from all corners of the hallway.

My doctor and I visited through my hiccups and cries, and he examined my rashes (that had nearly disappeared entirely). He said, "You look so much better, and I feel comfortable with you going home. I think there is a slim chance of these current symptoms being graft-versus-host, and you're already on a high dose of Prednisone. Also, I'll see you tomorrow for your appointment. We can get a stool sample then. Just call if there are any changes or more diarrhea." I told him he was my angel, and I felt so blessed to have such a fantastic doctor. There was a newfound trust that sprouted in our relationship that day. I am still in awe that he took the time to see me.

I immediately called my dad to see if he could come back and get me. Fortunately, he had just left the parking garage and was more than happy to turn around and wait until I had finished wrapping everything up at the hospital. The nurses gave me a unit of magnesium, and my dad and I headed back home – where I belong. Thank God!

I saw my doctor the next day and willingly supplied a stool sample. The results were negative for graft-versus-host. I have a strong feeling that the diarrhea was due to overeating the delicious soup and nothing more. Lesson learned: Be mindful of my serving size when reintroducing my body to food!

The past couple of days have resulted in some intense emotional whiplash... and it's times like these that the ratio between good and bad starts to scale in the wrong direction. It sucks when the bad feels too significant to move forward. I'm still working my way through the weeds, though! Soon enough, all the pests will be excavated, and I'll reveal the healthy, vibrant flowers that were here all along.

 Philippians 4:7 ~ And the peace of God, which transcends all understanding, will guard your hearts and your minds in Christ Jesus.

CANCER BE GONG!

Some people believe holding on and hanging in there are signs of great strength. However, there are times when it takes much more strength to know when to let go and then do it.

~ Ann Lander

Do you ever hold onto items you 'think' you might need someday, only to find yourself never going back to retrieve them? The basket of magazines in my family room, the stack of articles in my office – what I call a 'must-read later' pile that I seldom revisit. Why am I holding onto last year's news anyway? On the other hand, I keep some outdated items because they contain some esteemed 'value.' For example, Shaylee often writes me sweet messages on whatever scrap of paper she can find. I usually keep them tucked away because they mean something to me. But I have to admit that I don't find myself going through the notes to reread very often. Nonetheless, sometimes I stumble across one of Shayee's notes when I least expect it, and her messages happen to be precisely what I need at that moment.

You may be wondering where I'm going with this. Well, I had a revelation during my doctor's appointment on Tuesday, September 26, day thirty-eight post-transplant. I told my doctor that I had a CANcer box in my closet. It's devoted to countless papers of lab work dating years back, my hair clippings from when they shaved my head (both times), and miscellaneous items that I felt needed to be included. I even saved all my caps and wigs (which I ended up donating to the hospital for someone else in need).

Most of the illness items don't serve a purpose for my highest good. These unnecessary keepsakes have resided in that box for the full course of my disease, and after depositing more paperwork and mementos following each doctor's visit, not once do I dare to unfasten the lid and examine the collection inside. I'm not sure if I keep it tucked away to feign temporary healthiness or if I think it would be nice to look back on later in life, but that box of horrors definitely mocks me with the ugly memories stored within.

With my recurrence of leukemia, I began to realize that the box was not necessarily a bombshell of sadness – it also held the many reminders of blessings that showed up due to my CANcer. It was helpful to retrieve those meaningful items and take them with me during extended stays in the hospital.

Back to the point of this story, I continued to tell my doctor that I wanted to let go of CANcer in my own way. I planned on having a burning ceremony to dispose of all the things in the dreadful box that held no positive sentimental value. I'm only going to keep the "G.I. Mary Jane" banner and other small motivational items. For me, physically seeing the blemishes of my past erupt into flames will invoke a type of release that's unachievable in the office of a therapist. As of now, I'm still anchored to my leukemia. I want to float back to the surface and be known by more than just my health.

It's not that I want to erase my memories, but rather that I believe letting go with symbolic flames will free me from their weight. The only thing I had yet to figure out was the date I was going to ignite the fire. Then, my doctor said, "You should do it on the hundred-day celebration." Amen to that!

During my appointment, I found out that the graft-versus-host disease on my arms is clearing up beautifully and that I could get my PICC line removed! I've had the PICC line in since May 19 (a little over four months), and taking it out will mark another milestone.

Tim and I drove straight to the other clinic for the line removal. When we arrived, we were directed over to a small room, and the deed was done! After the procedure, the nurse led us to the sacred gong, titled "Cancer be Gong," and told me to hit it with a mallet. There were three mallets to choose from: big, medium, and small. Of course, I chose the biggest one! GONG!! What an enormous high it was to give it a good ole whack! The nurses and patients cheered for my accomplishment, and I had the biggest grin on my face. Things are 'gonging' in the right direction! My new life is beginning to come together.

1 Corinthians 9:24 ~ Do you not know that in a race all the runners run, but only one gets the prize? Run in such a way as to get the prize.

Day 50 of Isolation and a Homecoming

I can't believe I've reached the halfway mark to my one hundred days of isolation after my stem cell transplant. My blood work continues to look good, and my doctor said that everything is going accordingly. Yesterday, I was able to drop my Prednisone medication down to only ten milligrams a day, which is fantastic news! My body is less itchy, and I am pain-free. Food tastes delightful now, and I'm putting on some of the weight I lost after the transplant. I still need to work on my stamina, but I am grateful to be doing so well. A few days ago, I even began committing to a light exercise, sometimes walking for brief periods or engaging in a ten to fifteen-minute beginner's yoga workout. It was nothing too crazy or long-lasting, but I have to start somewhere! I need to find my 'new normal' again and am working toward uncovering it piece by piece.

Lately, it's been busy at the Robinson household with doctor appointments, lab work, and the kids' activities. One of the biggest highlights was the high school homecoming celebration that Brody and Holly attended last weekend. Of course, I would have loved to be the one to help both of them prepare for the event, but I couldn't go out in public. So Tim took Brody and Holly shopping, even though it was out of his comfort zone. Even though I couldn't participate in as much of the preparation process as I would have liked, I was just grateful to be here to witness them at the peak of their high school experience.

Here's to good health and longevity!

 Jeremiah 29:11-13 ~ "For I know the plans I have for you," declares the Lord, "plans to prosper you and not to harm you,

plans to give you hope and a future. Then you will call on me and come and pray to me, and I will listen to you. You will seek me and find me when you seek me with all your heart."

MOMENT OF TRUTH

The real winners in life are the people who look at every situation with an expectation that they can make it work or make it better.

~ Barbara Pletcher

It's already the end of October, and I'm on day sixty-four of my post stem cell transplant. I can't wait for this isolation phase to be over. The end of isolation doesn't mean immediate freedom, though. My doctor told me that even when the one hundred days were over, I would need to continue being careful around large crowds for quite some time. He followed up by saying it could take up to two years for my immune system to stabilize fully, but, of course, the first one hundred days are the most critical. At this point, I'll be fine as long as I can spend occasional time outdoors – anything is better than the confinement of my house.

A few days ago, I had another appointment with my herbalist. I firmly believe that his aid is vital to my overall recovery. I always gather blood work and other medical information from my doctor to make the most of our visits. Believe it or not, blood work provides a vast amount of helpful information about my body's natural function. And since I have lab work done so often, it's always interesting to see how much my results change in-between consultations.

At this appointment, my herbalist looked over my blood results from the most recent labs and talked briefly with me about how I had been feeling. Then he did his routine exam of traditional Chinese medicine (TCM). This practice includes a tongue exam, as, according to the principles of TCM, the tongue is a prime indicator of bodily health. My herbalist also utilizes a pulse examination (a diagnostic technique that checks pulse levels on the wrists). Both of these assessments were common demonstrations and practices in the Herbal Program I had started participating in last year. There was so much knowledge I had yet to acquire!

My herbalist is typically a man of few words during our consultations, but on this particular day, he asked if anything was bothering me. Apparently, my pulse diagnostics indicated that my heart was sad. I told him that sometimes I do feel sad. I get frustrated that I still don't have the energy I once had. But, I also had a sense of guilt because I should be rejoicing about how well I am doing right now. After all, I was in remission.

Clearly, I had been through a lot. Of course, there were inactive periods when I wasn't feeling well, but I don't think I realized how much they had affected me emotionally. I recalled the social worker (in charge of weekly meetings for leukemia and lymphoma patients at Nebraska Medicine) uses the term post-traumatic stress disorder (PTSD) for those who have had a stem cell transplant. And I suppose that makes sense... I'm never going to forget the pain I went through.

As my session came to a close, I waited for my custom-made herbal tincture in the waiting room. Then my herbalist approached me with a minimalist and sophisticated-looking card. It had a red ribbon tied through two holes on the top and exhibited three simple drawings on the front. Each drawing showcased some type of contentment: The first was a person laughing, the second was two individuals hugging each other with a heart above them, and the third was a person in a meditation position holding a yin-yang symbol. Beneath the pictures, the words "Do behavior that feeds your spirit" were artfully printed. Inside the card, my herbalist had also written a touching note. He said to live in spirit – inspiration; if I allow my spiritual inspiration to shine, miracles will follow.

After I left with my updated herbal tincture, I regretted not discussing *exactly* why he thought my heart was sad. Maybe it was something I needed to discover on my own? I suppose it could have been because I was in isolation at the time and was not seeing friends very often. It also could be from my loss of stamina or other subconscious insecurities. Most likely, it's a combination of both. All I know right now is that I need to find my true self again.

My herbalist did suggest that I purchase, *Love yourself, Heal Your Life Workbook* by Louise Hay. He insisted that it would help me heal areas in my life that I may not have even considered. Taking his recommendation seriously, I ordered a copy right away and began to skim through it. During my reading, my mind kept going back to, "What did *I* do to cause leukemia and for it to return?" I knew there was nothing I could have done – chromosome sixteen simply had a glitch – but I still feel like I should have done more to prevent it.

Some of the suggested affirmations were super helpful in realizing that no one is to blame for my suffering. I decided to make a list of the reminders that resonated with me most so I could refer back to them easily. Now, multiple times a day, I reaffirm that "I deserve life, a good life. I deserve the highest good. I am beautiful, bold, and courageous. I am healthy. I have total freedom and am willing to create new thoughts. I am strong and have a voice. I am everything that I need to be." The list goes on. Regular appreciation for ourselves shifts us into greater acceptance. I want to maximize my potential and be thankful for all that God has made me to be.

This book also helped me reflect on my inner child. I know this may seem strange to some, but as I wrote answers to the questions in the workbook, memories that I hadn't thought of in years came flooding back. Some of them brought a smile to my face, while others I would have preferred to have stayed buried. These experiences, as hard as they were to face, helped me establish a new outlook: I am finished with regrets. My past is simply the story of how I've reached my current self.

This realization calls for a session of forgiveness. I forgive those who have hurt me. And I forgive myself for my own mistakes – both the faults of my younger days and inevitable mess-ups that are sure to come in my future. Why are we living, if not to learn? I am grateful for every dumb decision and hasty experience I've endured.

We live in an imperfect world. Unfortunately, sometimes relationships and activities bring out our bad side. But becoming aware of toxicity is the first step toward a more grounded self. We can recreate our reality by adjusting our focus; this could mean distancing ourselves from draining friends and finding friends who compliment our best traits, or even quitting our job and finding something more suitable to our interests. Regardless, refocusing requires looking deeper into our hearts. Think about your passion. How can you utilize your spirit to accomplish that which you love?

Ebers Papyrus (one of the oldest medical documents of ancient Egypt) says that no disease can remain in the body when joy exists in the heart. I want a fulfilled life, and I will never stop exploring new methods to discover what satisfaction entails.

Heal Your Body A-Z by Louise Hay provides a list of new thought patterns through affirmations, "Joyous new ideas are circulating freely within me. I move beyond past limitations into the freedom of the now. It is safe to be me." Amen to those new thoughts! I claim all of them in Jesus' name.

 Proverbs 17:22 ~ A cheerful heart is good medicine, but a crushed spirit dries up the bones.

THROUGH THE EYES OF A CHILD

Pretty much all the honest truth-telling there is in the world is done by children.

~ Oliver Wendell Holmes

There are several times in a woman's life when she undergoes changes in her body. Menopause is one of the final transitions, and I began experiencing its symptoms at an earlier age than most. Starting in October, I have suffered from hot flashes multiple times a day and often throughout the night. Now it's the end of November, and the overwhelming heat has yet to cease.

One minute I'm fine, and the next, I'm burning up and sweating (needing to remove my head cap, fan myself, and take off layers of fabric). This sudden onset of warmth only lasts a minute or so, but it certainly affects my sleep during the night. I don't always talk about everything that my body goes through during my treatments, but this is one physical reaction I cannot hide. When the clothes or blankets need to come off, there's nothing stopping me, and my family just has to deal with it. Now that I have set the stage for my annoyances, here's the rest of the story:

A few days ago, Shaylee was outdoors shooting hoops with the basketball, riding the scooter, and running around with the dogs for quite some time. I told her that she needed to wear a coat because it's been pretty chilly outdoors lately. After a while, I heard Shaylee rushing into the house, throwing her coat off, and removing layers of clothing. She exclaimed, "Oh my gosh, I'm having a hot flash! I'm having a hot flash!" She fell to the floor and began fanning herself with the flannel shirt that was scrunched in her hand. Tim and I looked at each other, and all we could do was laugh. I guess this momma has been saying those words a lot lately, and perhaps I've been a bit overly dramatic about it. Little did I know, my ten-year-old daughter picked up on the struggle and thought hot flashes were simply from getting too warm! Naturally, we had a discussion about why I've had these sudden surges of intense heat lately, and now she understands the true meaning.

Although it's strange for me to undergo this 'change of life' at such a young age, I understand its reason. My body has gone through so much, and the treatments take a physical and mental toll. That doesn't mean that I can't see the humor in this situation with my daughter, though! Shaylee thinking she is having 'hot flashes' has also created a slight perspective shift in my thinking. Instead of seeing my menopause symptoms as unnatural and scary, perhaps I should treat them as an everyday experience. Adopting a normal attitude in a time when nothing feels normal might help me overcome the struggles.

Shaylee gave me a little gift when she flopped down on the floor with her 'hot flash.' Not only did she inspire wholehearted laughter, but she also boosted my self-reflection. I now know that my body is just doing what it needs to do in the given circumstances.

Recently, I haven't had to change my pajamas even once during the night! And I've barely sweated in my sleep for the past three days. Is it a coincidence? I think NOT! The miraculous happens when you embrace *what is*. Acknowledge the uncomfortable.

1 Thessalonians 5:16-18 ~ Rejoice always, pray continually, give thanks in all circumstances; for this is God's will for you in Christ Jesus.

DAY 100 OF ISOLATION AND FINAL BIOPSY

The journey between what you once were and who you are now becoming is where the dance of life really takes place.

~ Barbara De Angelis

The one-hundredth day of my isolation period finally arrived on November 30. Time to rejoice! I made it through the isolation phase intact. Even with this accomplishment, though, I hadn't forgotten about the conversation my doctor and I had on day thirty-eight about continuing to take things slow. I still had quite a ways to go before my immune system would return to its fully-functioning self. And as much as I wanted to burn the cancer box's items right now, I didn't have the ambition. The hundred-day mark sounds perfect on paper, but I'd rather wait until I felt less tired and weak. I wasn't mentally prepared to sift through the countless materials I had preserved over all those years. My soul will send an internal message when the time is right.

Now that I've reached the hundred days, I need one last bone marrow biopsy and aspiration to confirm that my body has accepted all of the donor's cells. Sure enough, the results showed that the male chromosomes in my DNA had finished their transition – the stem cell transplant was a success! My doctor phoned me personally to deliver this good news. He also mentioned that the preliminary tests showed that my blood type had changed to A positive, there was NO sign of leukemia, and everything was looking perfect. We will go over the rest of the results when they come in.

Wow, leukemia-free! I did it! I'm a winner! I can't explain what a relief that phone call was… in all my years of hoping, the confirmation of freedom was even more special than I imagined. I'm not even sure what to do at this point. I don't remember what it feels like not to be sick. My stem cell transplant is finally complete! Naturally, a tear-filled smile lingered on my face for days, exuding the joy from my grateful heart. God chose to save *me*.

But I can't be too quick to sing final praises – I'm not done with this fight quite yet. Despite the coming and going of the hundred days, my immune system is still weak. It could take as long as two years to stabilize everything that the stem cell transplant compromised. So, each day I pray - I pray for strength; I pray for faith; and I pray for everything to work out the way God intended.

 2 Samuel 22:33 ~ It is God who arms me with strength and keeps my way secure.

FIRST TIMES

Every experience is a once in a lifetime experience,
because no matter how hard we try,
nothing's ever exactly the same as it was the first time.

~ Jolene Perry

There is a first time for everything — a first smile… first word… first step… first dance… first kiss… first love. The list goes on and on. More often than not, these 'firsts' symbolize growth, providing foundations for expectations and values. For example, who could forget their first kiss? The contact simultaneously triggers emotional bursts in our brains and butterflies in our stomachs, opening our eyes to a whole new kind of companionship. Then, there's the first love – when it feels like the only two people on this planet are you and your partner, completely exposed and pure. And then all your priorities turn upside-down when your infant gives you that first gummy smile. It just warms your heart and somehow makes you love them even more. Then you get the privilege of watching your sweet child evolve in the same way you did – going to school, making friends, and moving on to a life of their own.

As beautiful as they seem, not every first is as delightful as the ones I've listed above. A recent not-so-enjoyable experience of mine was my first cardio workout since the stem cell transplant. I wasn't sure how my weakened body would react to this type of exercise, and after some experimentation, I can confidently say that I overestimated my vigor. My goal has been to *attempt* one workout video per day, disregarding my breathing struggles and inability to do most moves. As sad as it is, just making an effort to stand in front of the TV for twenty-five minutes a day seems to be helping my progress! Even so, for the past week, I've woken up with sore muscles and heavily-drained energy. Maybe I should tone it down even more notches. It's been challenging for me to find the right balance between exercise and rest – I often can't tell that I've overexerted myself until it's too late. Perhaps there's a delay in the communication between my body and mind. After spending so many months in a hospital bed, relearning my body's cues will definitely take some time.

Triggered by thoughts of transformation, an idea came to me. I remembered hearing about a revitalization program at the YMCA during my first battle with CANcer. It is called LiveSTRONG. This free (one-time) twelve-week group training program is designed specifically for cancer survivors. It's geared toward building strength, confidence, and physical endurance. I would have liked to participate back in 2015, but it never worked out. NOW feels like the perfect time to start.

I decided to call the local YMCA and ask if they offered LiveSTRONG at their location. As fate would have it, the receptionist said they just approved their first session ever, set to begin in early February. I hung up the phone excitedly and knew this group would be my saving grace. The nudge of team effort will inspire me to reach my fitness goals at a reasonable pace. I'm ready to PUMP IT UP!

LiveSTRONG will be another 'first' to check off my list, bringing me even closer to optimal health. Each of these firsts symbolizes steps into the wisdom of adulthood. Yes, some steps are steeper and less stable than others, but the stairway of life has one hell of a destination. There's still so much more for me to learn and see, but I can tell you one thing for certain: I recommend making that climb.

Romans 15:13 ~ May the God of hope fill you with all joy and peace as you trust in him, so that you may overflow with hope by the power of the Holy Spirit.

SWEAT IT OUT!

Every woman who heals herself helps heal all the women who came before her, and all those who come after her.

~ Dr. Christiane Northrup

In May, I attended a sweat lodge hosted by Native Americans. This opportunity came from my herbalist class. And although my instructor said that the special ceremony was not a requirement for our course, I happily signed up. I'd never done anything like it before, and a deep cleanse sounded like just the thing I needed! When I shared the fun news with my mother, her reaction wasn't as excited as expected. She shared a bit about how the lodges worked and warned me that the tipi became uncomfortably hot. My mom was a teacher on the Pine Ridge Reservation in South Dakota for many years, and although she had never desired to enter a sweat lodge, she was very familiar with their functions. Her notions made me slightly concerned about the high temperature conflicting with my stem cell transplant recovery, so I asked my instructor for his thoughts. Simply put, he said that if I felt compelled to go, I should.

And that's precisely what I did! Bring on the heat! Upon our arrival, each member of my class presented a gift to the medicine man of their tribe. We also brought along prayer ties to burn. A classmate and I had gotten together ahead of time and made our prayer ties by cutting bits of red cloth into small squares. We wrote our prayer requests on strips of paper, folded them into the fabric, and looped yarn around each bundle. The connected bundles formed a long chain.

When I pictured the sweat lodge session, I imagined silence and meditation, but the Native Americans brought mind-blowing energy. They played drums, chanted, and enthusiastically sang in their language. Between these jubilant chants and songs, each of us had an opportunity to express what was on our minds. Some of us asked for help; others prayed.

Regardless of what we were thinking, the lodge's power moved most of us to tears. When it was my turn to speak, I tossed my prayer bundle in the flaming-hot fire at the center of our circle group and pleaded for complete restoration. As the smoke rose to the top of the tipi-lodge and escaped through the small hole, I imagined all of my prayer requests releasing to heaven. I forgot all about the heat and could feel years of negative emotions seeping out of my body, dripping to the depths of the Earth. After the ceremony, everyone stepped outside the lodge to rehydrate with fruit, snacks, and drinks. The gentle outdoor breeze was refreshing since my entire body and clothing were drenched. Luckily, I brought a dry towel to wipe the remaining drops of sweat beads. It was an uncomfortable drive home, sitting in my wet clothes, but the healing benefits were so worth it!

My instructor shared a message from his former teacher: "When you learn Native ways, you learn to dance, sing, express, and cry." The sweat lodge was so much more than I thought it would be, and I enjoyed the session so much that my friend and I went to another ceremony at the same location the following week. Only this time, it was open to the public, so all sorts of people sat beside us. The large-group experience just meant I was a bit less vulnerable. Nonetheless, both experiences were powerful. Sometimes we need to reach our breaking point before we can let go of our burdens.

 Luke 22:43-44 ~ An angel from heaven appeared to him and strengthened him. And being in anguish, he prayed more earnestly, and his sweat was like drops of blood falling to the ground.

RANDOM ACTS OF KINDNESS

Each smallest act of kindness reverberates across great distances
and spans of time, affecting lives unknown to the one
whose generous spirit was the source of this good echo,
because kindness is passed on and grows each time it's passed,
until a simple courtesy becomes an act
of selfless courage years later and far away.

~ Dean Koontz

There is so much good in this world. The clouded lens of the media can sometimes convince us otherwise, but if we stop and look around, selflessness and compassion are everywhere. Have you ever given up your precious time to help a friend in need? Or paid for the person behind you in the drive-thru just because you were feeling generous? These temporary shifts in your priorities – asking for nothing in return and focusing on someone whose problems outweigh yours – are demonstrations of LOVE. Humans inherently love, and making time to care for one another is the driving force behind our species' survival. And this love wouldn't be possible without the foundation of trust. Your individual choice to show some love can trigger so many more acts of kindness and support.

It's December 29, and I recently received a mysterious package in the mail. The exterior was nothing out of the ordinary – a large, brown manila envelope with no return address or sender's name – but the interior blew me away. Enclosed was a women's devotional book, an angel pin, a beautiful one-page typed letter signed by *Anonymous*, and a generous monetary gift. This package was such a wonderful surprise, and it had arrived at the perfect time. I peeked inside the envelope again to search for clues, hoping to find even a speck of evidence that could hint at the sender's identity. Unfortunately, they were too clever for me, and my search left me with no more information than what I had started with. I so desperately wanted to thank this kind soul for their thoughtful and selfless deed, but I guess acts of love really do mean the person wants nothing in return. All I could do was look up to the heavens with tear-filled eyes and thank God for my blessings.

This generosity reminded me of the "Giving to the Needy" story in the book of Matthew. It states: "Be careful not to practice your righteousness in front of others to be seen by them. If you do, you will have no reward from your Father in heaven. So when you give to the needy, do not announce it with trumpets, as the hypocrites do in the synagogues and on the streets, to be honored by others. Truly I tell you, they have received their reward in full. But when you give to the needy, do not let your left hand know what your right hand is doing, so that your giving may be in secret. Then your Father, who sees what is done in secret, will reward you."

The anonymous donor's 'secret service' came with no accolades, no thank-yous, and no recognition. Or did it somehow? I believe this Bible passage conveys that even when we aren't acknowledged for our good deeds by others, God still notices them and rewards us in unexpected ways. We need to stop missing the point of giving – helping others is not an excuse to put the spotlight on ourselves.

Of course it's nice to be praised and appreciated, but Matthew's Bible verse reminds us that we need only to delight God. Perhaps you should check your motives from time to time and ask yourself, "What would Jesus do? And why would Jesus do it?" My mysterious gift-giver must be wise beyond their years. Sometimes I even struggle with the idea of being purely kind (no ulterior motives).

After reading the anonymously-written letter several times, I began to think of ways *I* could help others – even if it's just with a simple phone call to check in on an old friend or choosing to open the door for a stranger. Kindness doesn't have a price tag; there are so many ways we can help each other. Additionally, science has proven that selflessness blesses *all* individuals involved. Research shows that giving and receiving kindness is beneficial for the body. It can reduce stress and improve physiological function. I hope my secret sender knows how humbled I am to receive their act of love. Maybe one day, they will have the opportunity to read my story and realize how much of an impact they've made.

As I glimpse into my past, I realize that this package wasn't my only anonymous gift. The precious stem cells that saved my life were also given to me by an anonymous donor. However, in this case, they were from a complete stranger. Perhaps we can all aspire to give a little more in life – you never know how much it can change someone's life.

Colossians 3:12 ~ Therefore, as God's chosen people, holy and dearly loved, clothe yourselves with compassion, kindness, humility, gentleness and patience.

RISKY MOVES

I am thankful for all of it. The highs. The lows. The blessings.
The lessons. The setbacks. The comebacks. The love. The hate.
Everything. They are what got me to be where I am today,
and I am proud of where I am today.

~ Unknown

On February 4, 2018, the sermon at church was: Don't *ask why*. That's a tough order to follow sometimes, right? It's difficult not to question God's plan when it feels like *we* are the only ones who truly know what's best for our wellbeing. But that's okay; a bit of rebellion is natural, and, ultimately, our downfalls help us realize how dependent we really are on God's saving grace. Once on His destined course, your growth will create new pathways to even greater goals. Stop holding yourself back and embrace His design! All you need to do is establish a relationship of trust with Him – enough trust to eliminate all possibilities of doubt. Again, I know that this is no easy task (believe me, I'm still working on it), but consider all that God has sacrificed for us to live freely. He offers us the world and asks for nothing more than our obedience and love in return. That's a pretty decent trade, if you ask me.

Going back to the sermon itself, I've had difficulty with 'not questioning God' for the past couple of months. It's hard not to ask "why" when my fingernails proceed to fall off and my skin won't stop peeling. Is my suffering His intention? Did God really plan for my life to end in this way? I now realize that His trials taught me perseverance, strength, and patience, but I'll admit it: I was angry about His choices back then. No one deserves to go through the kind of pain and horror that I underwent. Nonetheless, God has His own way of opening our eyes to that which we refuse to see. He knew that I could handle it, and I am glad to be out on the other side.

Lately, my family has really enjoyed playing card games. *Pitch* is a family favorite. When it's time to play, we gather around the table to share laughs, make connections, and appreciate some fun competition. I won't go into too much detail regarding *Pitch's* ins and outs, but I'll cover some basic rules to enhance overall understanding. Whoever is the first one to collect a total of fifty-two points wins the game. Each round, a hand has the potential to earn its wielder and their partner ten points. At the beginning of the matches, each family member will have a chance to call out their bid, declaring how many points they *think* they can collect. The highest bidder gets to choose the suit! Sometimes, the bidder earns their predicted points with no problem at all. Other times, meeting the bid can be a much bigger struggle. It's always comical when one of us fails so much that our points start to dive into the negative values!

Now that you know most of the technicalities, *Pitch* boils down to one key strategy – shooting the moon! During a bid, this call is an option that means a person thinks they can collect ALL ten of the potential points. And they put everything on the line for that play. What makes it so risky is that if the person fails to gain the ten points as they had claimed they would, their point value will drop back down to zero. Failure to shoot the moon basically ruins your likelihood of victory, but when done properly, the shooter who earns all ten points will automatically win and end the game early. Pretty powerful move, huh? Tim is usually the one in our family to shoot the moon – he has always been a thrill-seeker. And, annoyingly, his risk usually pays off! Tim wins the most out of all of us. Hmm… maybe there is something to this risk-taking thing.

I have never been a natural risk-taker, but I have recently learned that sometimes calculated gambles can pay off in a big way. I don't have to shoot the moon every time, but being open to its possibility has helped improve my awareness and overall strategy. I suppose the point is that we can't shut down options simply because we're afraid of them. Sometimes making a 'scary move' is the only way to win the game.

I met my goal! My doctors recently took me off of my anti-rejection medication six months post-transplant, I decided it might finally be time to start living a little. I'm ready for those calculated risks! Being in isolation for so long put me in desperate need of a change of scenery. Upon clearing it with my doctor, I decided to fly to Arizona with my mom to visit my brother Matt. I had specific instructions to wear thick layers of sunscreen and stay clear of germs. I brought the sunscreen recommended for stem cell transplant patients, a container of antibacterial wipes, masks, and rubber gloves. Now I'm ready to take on anything! The flight to Phoenix was pleasant, and I took advantage of the time to rest.

Mom and I didn't have plans to do much while there, other than to enjoy the warm weather and, of course, spend quality time with Matt. But Matt, being the way he is, had different plans for us. Even though I was hesitant about his agenda (because it meant that I would need to be among crowds), I decided to be bold and just roll with the punches. I couldn't live in a bubble for the rest of my life.

During the day, Matt gave mom and me a tour of the local museums and introduced us to some of his favorite eateries. In the evening, he grilled delicious meals at his home while my mom and I rested. After all, we had to prepare ourselves for the next day's adventure! He treated us like royalty.

The trip went on to be the best decision ever, and Matt provided several more entertaining activities for mom and me to enjoy. I got a real taste of what Arizona has to offer! One of my most memorable highlights was ziplining. The simultaneous thrill and fear of zooming down the cable made me feel like a kid again – the height of the starting point was impressive in itself. Matt and I were carted high up into the mountains, and the view from the landing platform seemed to go on forever. Below us lay a deep valley filled with dried dirt and cacti. I looked up and realized that only a metal cable and sketchy pulley would lie between us and instant death. I crossed my fingers and prayed that Matt and I would make it to the bottom unscathed. It was too late to back out now. So, we did the only thing we could do and jumped forward. Our rapid descent down the cable awakened a feeling of freedom I didn't even know existed. We shrieked and laughed at the mere absurdity of it all – we were FLYING. If you had asked me a few years ago, I wouldn't have seen much logic in a dangerous activity like ziplining. Now I see the beauty in its risk.

Matt and I paid extra for a GoPro photo that was automatically taken while we were shooting down the zipline. Our mouths were wide-open in screams, our hair was slicked back, and our arms were around each other. I was so grateful to have shared this frightening adventure with my brother. And our mom had the pleasure of watching the magic from the sidelines.

After the zipline, Matt took us to an outdoor restaurant with live country music. Folks were line dancing and having a great time. I've always wanted to line dance, and so I got up and joined them. It felt so good to get out of my shell a bit – even if I occasionally messed up the moves. I've always loved dancing and even took ballet, tap, and jazz lessons for several years as a child. I still have the costumes from all the dance recitals that I participated in, and my girls loved to dress up in the sequinned leotards when they were younger. Sweet memories continued to rush back as I continued my line dance indulgence on the dance floor.

Riding on Matt's Harley Davidson bike took me back in time again, too. I hadn't ridden on a motorcycle in years. It was so liberating – the warm sun on my face, a gentle breeze tickling my skin, and the music blasting from the Harley's stereo. Nothing could wipe the smile off my face! When we returned to Matt's house, I called Tim and said we absolutely *needed* to go motorcycle-riding when I got back home. I didn't know that I would enjoy myself so much!

I've started to realize that pushing ourselves outside of our comfort zone is good for our souls. During this trip, I was reminded of the refreshment of youth and free spirit. My sickness and seriousness seem to have made me lose sight of those luxuries. I became frightened to go out into the world. I was stuck worrying about germs, sun exposure, and triggering graft-versus-host disease. Matt helped me remember what it's like to have fun again. The risk that came with visiting Arizona was well worth it.

Unfortunately, amid all of the wonders of life, I have also recently had some sobering moments. I have lost eight friends this year – all of whom received stem cell transplants around the same time as I did. One loss, in particular, was difficult for me to process. One day, I found myself scrolling through the latest news on Facebook, and I saw that my former hairstylist had another baby boy. I was so happy for her. To provide a little background, she had been my hairstylist for several years, so our life updates every few months were always packed with conversation. She has three boys, and it was pretty common for us to share laughs about the joys of children. Her haircuts were rejuvenating in more ways than just the service.

In 2015, her youngest son was diagnosed with acute myeloid leukemia. It sank my heart. I couldn't believe that this young, healthy, vibrant child had contracted the same illness as me. She ended up taking time off work to take care of her son. When he reached remission, she returned to the salon, and I continued coming back to her for haircuts. We visited about his condition and the general surprise of his leukemia. Just like me, there was no family history. Unfortunately, her son's leukemia relapsed as the months went on, and he needed a stem cell transplant from a donor. If my memory serves me correctly, he was in remission for about eight months. I was so sad for their family. About three months after his cancer crept back, mine had too.

When I saw her on Facebook with her new baby, I was so excited! I decided to read more. As I scrolled down to see how her other son was doing after his stem cell transplant, I discovered that he passed away from a terrible infection in September of 2017. His death looked to be due to complications from pneumonia, his immune system being too depleted to fight back. I had no idea.

While I was receiving intensive chemo for remission in the hospital, he was on the opposite side of the hallway preparing for the stem cell transplant. Our paths crossed from time to time in the confined walls of the hospital, his mother and I exchanging brief updates on progress whenever we met. I occasionally peeked into his hospital room to say hello and offer my best wishes. Typically, he was happily playing on an electronic device and replied with a quick "Hi," eager to get back to his game. He looked good, and that's the way I'd like to remember him.

I guess I was focused on making it through each day in my own battle and lost touch with others along the way. I felt so sorry for her family but also happy for the birth of her new son. I pray for blessings of peace as they journey ahead. It's moments like these that remind me of the preciousness of life. At first, I asked God (through tears), "Why?" What makes one person's outcome so different from others?

That lingering question brought me back again to the sermon: *Don't ask why*. We all process grief in different ways, but it somehow always ends the same – with acceptance. Instead of wasting our energy trying to figure out why things happen, trust in God's judgments. Instead of asking why, try asking, "What can I learn from this?" God's plan has bits of wisdom built in along the way, providing us with all that we need for fulfillment.

I can confidently say that He provided for me. God gave me the courage to make some risky moves! I shot the moon and won the game of life!

Proverbs 3:5-6 ~ Trust in the Lord with all your heart and lean not on your own understanding; in all your ways submit to him, and he will make your paths straight.

THE POWER OF WORDS

Nothing hurts a good soul and a kind heart more
than to live amongst people who cannot understand it.

~ Ali ibn Abi Talib

They say that time heals all wounds, but does it really? How can we patch up the wounds that we cannot see? Broken hearts, weary souls, and toxic environments leave lasting impressions. And, sometimes, the most we can do is learn how to adapt and live alongside these hardships.

It's May 7, and my mind has been racing the past few weeks. I've been thinking quite a bit about these internal scars... traumas I wish I could just forget. I would like to think that these denials are not exclusive to only me – all of us carry our own burdens. One of my first real memories of mental anguish was when my grandfather passed away. I was only ten years old when my mom received the devastating phone call. His death was so sudden – a heart attack just a day after my brother's twelfth birthday – and none of us were ready to grieve. Grandpa was the best, and at the time, it was difficult for me to cope with the fact that I would never see him again. I didn't know what to do with my sorrow except to cry. So, I sat uselessly on the couch with tears rolling down my cheeks, and there was no one there to comfort me. My brother told me to stop crying, and I obeyed. That day, I began suppressing my emotions, feeding into an unhealthy habit that stuck with me into adulthood. My grandpa's funeral came and went, and life moved on.

A year later, my dad accepted a teaching position at a college on the opposite side of Nebraska. It was so sad to leave the newly-finished house that my dad built from the ground up. I wasn't sure that I was ready for a new life – I loved my parochial school and amazing friends. After all, I was in the middle of fifth grade and had been there since kindergarten. My last day at this school was unbelievably special. The only downside was that the support of my teachers and classmates made it all the harder to leave. They had decided to throw me a surprise party, decking the classroom with cookies and other sweet refreshments. And it got even better than that! A stuffed teddy bear wearing a white sweatshirt sat in the center of the party. On the back of the sweatshirt were handwritten signatures from each student, leaving me with something to remember them by. My classmates told me that I could give the bear a tender squeeze whenever I needed the comfort of home. I cried when it was time to leave, and I wasn't sure that I would ever be ready for the challenge of public school in this unfamiliar town.

My mom and I drove over six hours to reach my dad and brother, who were already settled into our new home. With each mile, I held tighter onto that teddy bear, sometimes soaking its soft fur with stray tears. Once we arrived in this small college town, I did my best to put on a happy face. I wasn't accustomed to making new friends and wondered if I would fit in. Fortunately, on my first day of school, a small group of girls graciously accepted me into their circle. Their kindness helped fill the void in my heart.

I made it through the rest of fifth grade and most of sixth grade with no trouble, but the end of sixth grade came with some challenges. My people-pleasing tendencies pressured me to worry about everyone else's happiness, so I always pushed myself to be the perfect girl. This 'bending-over-backward' to make everyone happy attracted quite a bit of attention, and I started getting noticed by other groups of kids. As a result, I slowly shifted my concentration to a different set of friends. With these popular kids, I found myself creeping into activities that weren't true to my nature. They pushed me into the role of a follower, not a leader. I yearned for acceptance and approval so much that I didn't lead with my intuition, making the mistake of leaving behind the friends that were so kind to me when I first arrived. I was a lost soul trying to find my way into a place of belonging.

My facade continued into seventh grade, and the school's yearly talent show was approaching. My friend group had formed a dance team, and although we went through with the performance, we were all on each other's last nerve. One girl, in particular, criticized my every move and always made sure to highlight my mistakes. It was not a fun activity. Shortly after the show, a classmate handed me a thick note on my way to the next class. Back then, we wrote notes, folded them up real small, and sneakily delivered them to their recipient. There was a sense of thrill in receiving a message. So, when I got settled in my next class, I hastily unfolded the piece of paper and did my best to keep it hidden from my teacher and classmates. I focused on the bold words at the top of the multi-paged letter: 40 THINGS I HATE ABOUT MARY. I sank a bit lower in my seat and held back tears as I read: 1. Mary is always hungry. 2. She thinks she has to eat something all the time. 3. ALWAYS. The list went on and on, but I had to stop reading it in class, as I was on the brink of a panic attack.

I quickly folded the note and tucked it safely away until I got home, where I could sit alone and finish reading it. I was devastated... the girls whom I thought were my friends had abandoned me. Cruel insults were one thing, but forty of them? To know that people hated me so extensively made me feel worthless, and my insecurity only grew. I was too embarrassed to talk to my parents about it, so I opened a shoebox from my closet and set the note inside, pretending it never happened. Just another internal wound added to my soul.

Things did not improve as I moved into the following year. In eighth grade, a rumor was started that I padded my bra with tissue paper. Kids called me "Paddy" and always asked me for a tissue when passing by in the halls. It sounds ridiculous that I was so upset about this now (as an adult), but at that time, I was humiliated and frantic. I had always been sensitive, and my feelings got hurt easily. One person's comment would fester into endless overthinking and confusion. What did I need to change to make people like me? I was being attacked by false accusations, and there was nothing I could do about it. Both the boys and the girls in my class teased me endlessly. It got to the point that I had to go to the school counselor every day during lunch and recess, hoping for some fragment of relief. The counselor had discussions with some of the 'ring leaders,' but nothing seemed to help. The internal wounds began to pile on top of each other, and I was afraid my body was reaching maximum capacity.

After dealing with everything on my own for over a year, I decided to open up to my parents. I refused to mention the specifics of the harassment, but I broke down and cried to them nearly every night of eighth grade, begging them to let me live with my aunt or cousins in a different town. I even went to the effort of faking illnesses to miss school. I did everything I could to hang on to the little bit of light I had left in my heart. I'm honestly not sure how I made it through the school year in one piece. My depression was off the charts.

The teasing ended up fizzling out over summer break, and I discovered who my real friends were. I kept telling myself that things would be better in high school. As Mahatma Gandhi says, "You can't change how people treat you or what they say about you. All you can do is change how you react to it."

Over time, I built up a wall of protection. I was never going to let people see the hurt in me again. My middle school days were behind me. Of course, this strength was all for show, but my anxiety was so severe that I had nothing else to lean on. The only thing I could think to do was resort back to my people-pleasing tendencies. I had gotten myself stuck in a cycle of self-sabotage. My heart was hardened, and my true identity was lost.

That summer, I was introduced to alcohol and cigarettes by some peers. Unfortunately, this indulgence spiraled into a weekend routine, sometimes occurring even more frequently than that. It was a way to escape past pain, regrets, and misfortunes. Drinking helped me mute those 'internal wounds,' concealing what I wasn't ready to accept. I had finally found a way to bypass perfection.

Sadly, alcohol became a crutch, hindering my spiritual growth and family bonds. Fortunately, although it took me a few more years to realize it, I slowly realized that this lifestyle was holding me back and shifted to more responsible activities.

For as long as I can remember, I've found comfort in writing. Giving a voice to my feelings helps me cope in a way that nothing else can. As a young child, I would bring a notebook and pen to my brother's extra-curricular activities and write whatever came to mind. Jotting thoughts down on paper gave me the freedom to express myself without worries of judgment, ridicule, or competition. Writing also granted me time to reflect and recognize the parts of myself that I needed to focus on.

The social aspect of school wasn't always easy, but it taught me so much about myself and others. I wish I had avoided drinking and smoking entirely, but I feel like I also learned from those mistakes. It's best not to dwell on the choices of our pasts. There is no getting around childhood struggles. And I think that Maya Angelou gives some exceptionally-relevant advice: "Do the best you can until you know better. Then when you know better, do better."

Now that I think about it, I wonder if there's something to my 'faking' illnesses to get out of school when I was younger. Could my subconscious mind recall this as a way to get out of uncomfortable situations? I certainly hope not, but I also realize that (as an adult) for several years, there was a lot of tension in my office at work, and I chose to endure it for too long. Our department issues were never adequately resolved. Ultimately, most of my life has been filled with too much pressure. And no one is to blame for that but me. Perhaps the leukemia's BIG punch in the face was my body's way of removing myself from stress and toxicity. Now I have a better understanding of what we can bring upon ourselves with negative thought patterns. The rebirth of my stem cell transplant gave me a chance to start anew.

As for the "40 things I hate about Mary" note… Well, a few years back, Tim and I had plans of finishing our basement with the addition of another kitchen, bedroom, and family room area. I was sorting through boxes to get rid of items we no longer needed and happened to stumble across the shoebox of my past. Inside were various photos of me with friends, love letters from past flames, and other miscellaneous treasures acquired over the years. Among those cherished items were the folded-up pages from seventh grade. I had forgotten that I kept that dreaded note.

Slowly, I opened it and reread the silly reasons for hating me. I felt stupid for letting this note consume me so much back then and decided its existence was not for my highest good. Why did I prolong my suffering? I tore it up immediately and chucked it into the trash. Good riddance! Perhaps I should have burned it instead. The only good that came out of it was that I was able to understand and help my children if they ever had concerns about school bullies. Funny, maybe some of my 'so-called' past afflictions are actually teaching tools and blessings in disguise.

Interestingly enough, I recently came across another note tucked away in my desk, enclosed in a bright pink CD case. It was a surprise gift that I received in my mid-thirties from a good friend. Carefully, I opened the case. Inside, a neatly-folded piece of paper rested on top of a decorated CD (two photos of me alongside the words "Mary Jane's Last Dance" and "Mrs. Robinson" were printed on its face). The gift was just oozing love. I gently grasped the folded paper and peeked at the words inside. Upon seeing it again, I still couldn't believe what was written on the homemade, colorful stationery:

10 Things I Love About Mary

1. Her smile lights up a room.
2. She has a cute little laugh.
3. She can say anything with just her eyes!
4. Her legs are to die for!
5. I love how she wants everyone to like her.
6. I love that she is a sweet and caring friend that you can always count on and can always talk to... and the list went on.

She had no idea of the hateful note of my past and somehow knew exactly what to say to melt my heart. I played my friend's personalized CD and sang along to its sweet lyrics, fully unleashing my wild side. Then, I looked up to heaven and thanked God for her beautiful soul. Her act of kindness meant more to me than she would ever know. Notes of compassion are the only ones that matter.

 2 Corinthians 12:10 ~ That is why, for Christ's sake, I delight in weaknesses, in insults, in hardships, in persecutions, in difficulties. For when I am weak, then I am strong.

THE BOND OF FAMILY

One day someone is going to hug you so tight
that all of your broken pieces stick back together.

~ Anonymous

Cancer is not an exclusive illness. This is not to say that it's contagious or brings about other diseases, but rather that cancer impacts more than just the person with the diagnosis. Let me elaborate with an example: The minute the word "cancer" came out of my doctor's mouth, it immobilized all my plans and priorities, including those of my loved ones. In my case, I wasn't able to cook for my kids because I had to be in the hospital, so my friends took time out of their busy lives to donate meals. Additionally, I couldn't work in my condition, so the school district needed to find a temporary replacement. The 'strawberry jam' of cancer's presence, so to speak, spreads to the very edges of our bread piece, often spilling over the sides. And when we try to clean it up, we can't help but get our fingers sticky. From there, everything we touch is left with a translucent, gummy residue that refuses to wash off. Our life leaves a mark, and adding cancer to the mix can make things very messy. Again, cancer is not an exclusive illness. Everyone in our lives feels the pain alongside us.

I remember when my brother Matt came to visit for a few days before I got my stem cell transplant. It was a tense time for me, and I was constantly preoccupied with worries about the future. Most of our time spent together was over dinner, and it was nice to share memories while enjoying a warm meal. As one of these evenings came to a close, I headed to bed, thinking everyone else would too. It wasn't long before I heard obnoxiously-loud laughter coming from the other room. Although it typically would have been fine, I was tired, anxious, and needed to rest. So, I grudgingly rolled out of bed and told Matt and Tim that they were making it impossible for me to sleep – they either had to tone it down or go to bed. Expecting them to crumble under the weight of my ultimatum, I was surprised when Matt countered my annoyance with a less-agreeable reply. He said, "Mary, we are just letting out some steam and having fun. You know you aren't the only one going through this. It's affecting all of us."

Wow, that remark punctured my heart! Matt was absolutely correct. Yes, I was the one suffering through the painful and unpredictable treatments, but I couldn't forget that my loved ones were watching from the sidelines, cheering me on. I wonder how much emotion they have suppressed to preserve those happy faces. How much have they given up to ensure my smooth recovery?

As I contemplated Matt's comment even further, memories of the past came rushing back. I recall playing 'house' when I was a child. I would pretend to feed my doll, change soiled diapers and clothing, give baths, and take special care of her – that is, when I didn't forget about her and leave her in the corner for days. It was nice to have the option of not taking care of her if I didn't feel like playing anymore. My friends and I loved talking about the number of children we were planning on having and what their names would be. It was fun to dream about our Prince Charmings and happily ever afters.

Life was simple in my early years. There were no concerns about when the next meal was coming or if I would meet deadlines in time. I was free to be a kid, conquering any challenge that my imagination could conjure up. Eventually, though, I grew up and had *real* children. As precious as they are, I quickly learned that babies are much different from the dolls I used to play with – they need care every minute of every day. Newborns are not a piece of property that can be 'set in a corner' until you're in the mood to take care of them again. And even in their small state, babies have thoughts and feelings of their own. They need nurture and guidance. Being a parent is anything but easy. Nonetheless, the reward of being involved in every phase of your child's life is unimaginable.

Many people have inquired about how my children have dealt with my second diagnosis and slow recovery after the stem cell transplant. I always reply with, "As well as can be expected, considering all they have been through." Sometimes, I wish I could keep them in a protective bubble, eliminating all risks and concerns. But let's be honest, sheltering children too much may not be in their best interest either. Tim and I have done our best to be as open as possible with our kids, allowing them the freedom to express thoughts and feelings without having to fear consequences. Situations can get out of control, and I would always prefer that they ask for help instead of trying to go through challenges on their own.

I am grateful for the unbreakable bond of my family, especially that of my children. They are each blessed with unique personalities and strengths. Brody has a great sense of humor and an upbeat personality. Although he doesn't spend as much time with the family now that he's older, he's still my protector (just as my brother has always been). Brody likes to check in on me after coming home from work and outings – arms open, ready for a hug. I love it when he asks about my day and shares particulars about his.

He has such a sweet way of letting me know that he genuinely cares. I will always love his kind, compassionate heart.

Similar to Brody, Colby is also very protective of me. He's such a big helper and is always ready to complete whatever tasks I give him. And the best part is that Colby takes pride in his accomplishments, always eager for the compensation of hugs and enthusiastic praise. I love his passion and wit. My clever boy never turns down competitions or chances to showcase his skills. Even though Colby and Shaylee have had a few sibling quarrels, he is an excellent older brother. It's crazy that only a few minutes after a big argument, they're somehow always able to pick it right back up as if nothing had happened. I often see the two of them shooting hoops, riding the golf cart together, and exploring the outdoors.

Holly is taking the stresses of everyday life well, it seems. She is a girl of high standards and persistent efforts. With the widest array of interests in my family, she loves taking the stage in theatre, competing in tennis, playing intricate piano pieces, and assuming the role of a leader. And on top of all that, she is never seen without a good book. As I look back on Holly's prior year, it saddens me to think about all the extra responsibilities put on her when I was in the hospital and working through recovery. As with everything else, she was amazing at helping Tim with the two younger kids, doing laundry, tidying up the house, and preparing meals for everyone (when needed). I honestly have no idea how she was able to balance these additional tasks with the demands of her honors classes and extracurriculars. Holly took on so many things that a child her age should never have to worry about, and although she doesn't show it, I'm sure this secretly took a toll on her. Her diligence is what kept our family's puzzle interlocked, and, for that, I am eternally grateful.

Shaylee has always loved every minute of life. She is funny, great with animals, and cheerful in all her endeavors. I often see her running around outdoors with our dogs or cats, singing and laughing while inventing new activities for all of them to do. Shaylee enjoys arts and crafts and takes any opportunity to play with her older siblings. She is also incredibly smart, making inquiries about every little thing that crosses her path. In her younger years, Shaylee was extremely shy. She shrunk back from social settings and hid behind me while being introduced to new people. Fortunately, Shaylee has grown out of her bashful stage and appears to enjoy many friendships.

Having said all of that, I was a bit alarmed by Shaylee's demeanor when I told her that my CANcer had returned. She didn't show much expression on her face and went about her day as usual. I had concerns, but she assured me all was well. As I reflect on Shaylee's fourth-grade year, she seemed to be handling everything just fine, so I thought that perhaps there was nothing to worry about. However, as the school year progressed, Shaylee began showcasing signs of worry and anxiety. In the spring of that school year, April 24, 2018, I received a call from the school's secretary saying, "Shaylee has a bad stomach ache and is crying." So, I came and picked her up. She was perfectly normal and lively when we got home. I'm sure the chocolate shake, roast beef sandwich, and curly fries helped too! I had figured that maybe she was just hungry, but then the truth came out. Shaylee said she was really worried about the orchestra concert scheduled for that evening. The elementary students were supposed to take the bus to the middle school to practice beforehand, and the change in her after-school routine was nerve-racking. She had actually made herself sick from nerves. I felt terrible that she was so distressed over such small events. I can't say that her fears stemmed from my illness, but I'm sure my underlying poor health didn't ease her apprehensions.

Shortly after this first episode, Shaylee developed a habit of crying whenever I attempted to drop her off at school. She would consistently complain that her stomach hurt or that she didn't feel well. There was no coaxing her into staying, and so, each time, we went home. Upon returning home, Shaylee played with the dogs outside and acted fine for the rest of the day.

When I tried to take her back to school in the following days, the tears fell again and, suddenly, her stomach hurt. I was alarmed because this was very unlike Shaylee – I didn't understand what was happening. Her behavior was starting to give me déjà vu to when I had feigned illnesses in my challenging middle school years. I decided it was time to contact the school to see if they had noticed any unusual behavior. They said that they hadn't seen anything out-of-the-ordinary. Perplexedly, I asked them to keep a watchful eye on her because I was worried.

The emotional breakdowns became more frequent and more severe as the days went on. Shaylee began to cry for the entire twenty-minute drive to school. The car ride was heartbreaking, but I couldn't let her stay home if there was no reason. Most days, I had to walk her into the school's office and leave Shaylee in her sobbing and pleading state. It was horrible to see my daughter upset like this, and I so badly wished I could understand where her alligator tears were coming from. Occasionally, her fits would get the best of me, and I would yield, letting her come back home with me.

Both Tim and my other children were beginning to show frustration at Shaylee staying home from school so often. They thought it wasn't fair that she got so many unexcused breaks. I think they would have a different opinion if they saw how distraught she was whenever I tried to drop her off. I just couldn't bear leaving her at school so upset. I would sometimes cry right alongside Shaylee or weep alone during my drives home. Other times, I would get angry and lash out at her, questioning why she couldn't just stop crying! On those days, I felt terrible about how I handled it. I think my frustration was a defense mechanism of my own, trying to cover up my insecurity of being unable to help her as a mother. I desperately wanted my child back to her usual perky self.

As I mentioned earlier, Shaylee reminded me of what I went through in middle school; I understand the difficulty of not knowing how each day would play out. Even with this understanding, though, it felt like some of Shaylee's pieces were slowly disappearing from my family's puzzle. I needed to do something about it before she lost her place. So, it came time that I had to sit her down and fish out the real reason behind her outbursts.

Unfortunately, extracting Shaylee's thoughts was easier said than done. She wouldn't open up about anything, so I took her to my herbalist for help. He made a customized herbal tincture and provided suggestions on how to make Shaylee most comfortable in our home environment. She got to decorate her room with some new succulent plants and a miniature water fountain to soothe her mind.

All I could do from there was continue communicating with the school personnel and wait for any more behavior changes. Eventually, I got a call telling me that Shaylee had spoken with the school counselor. Shaylee told her about our dog Clyde, who had passed away right when I left for the hospital in August 2017. Honestly, I was surprised to hear about her hardship. Then, I remembered that I hadn't even talked to the kids about Clyde's death – and neither had Tim. We were too busy at the time, so

Tim decided to bury the dog on our acreage without the kids. Talk about sweeping the problem under the rug!

Immediately our family had a conversation about Clyde, and Shaylee said she regretted not being there more for him before he got sick and died. She was also sad that she didn't have the opportunity to say goodbye. Although we couldn't change what had happened, Tim and I decided that a ceremony for Clyde would help everyone process the loss a bit better. Shaylee picked out beautiful mums for his burial site, and we planted them so that his spirit could live on in nature. It gave us all closure.

Clyde's death felt symbolic of my latest cancer experience. I think Shaylee might be scared to lose me – perhaps all these changes are happening too quickly for her to process. It's clear now that I need to focus more on how my family is doing and less on my own concerns. My health is stable, but their mental states could be forever tarnished. I hope and pray that Shaylee begins to open up more.

 John 15:13 states, "Greater love has no one than this: to lay down one's life for one's friends." May Clyde rest in peace.

UNVEILING MORE TRUTHS

The hardest part of being a parent
is watching your child
go through something really tough
and not being able to fix it for them.

~ Anonymous

Shortly after Clyde's ceremony, I wrote a health update on CaringBridge, including a summary of how my children were doing and adding a brief account of Shaylee's recent struggles. I was so thankful when I received a text in response to my post from a previous colleague. She is a former counselor from the school district and works at a community family counseling practice in town. She thought it would be helpful if Shaylee visited with her at the counseling office. I was so grateful for her offer and scheduled an appointment right away.

I accompanied Shaylee during introductions and then stepped out of the room to give her privacy. When the counselor and Shaylee had finished visiting, I was brought back into the room. I had hoped that the space from her mother made her feel comfortable enough to share some of those pent-up feelings. With Shaylee's consent, we discussed some of the topics they addressed in her session. The counselor said that Shaylee didn't want to go to school anymore. She had mentioned that she felt "ignored" (her words) by her classmates. Some girls had been saying mean things that hurt her feelings, and she didn't have a lot of friends.

I also discovered that some classmates had been dumping her lunchbox out during lunchtime. They would search for the daily written note of encouragement (that I wrote to lift Shaylee's spirits) and read it aloud, laughing and passing it around. Another child would walk up to Shaylee's desk during art class and erase some of the drawings she was working on, saying that they were terrible. Recess was another brutal attack, as some kids wouldn't let her play on specific playground equipment and would exclude her from their games. I had no idea that any of this was going on. She never said a word to me about kids teasing her. Again, it reminded me of some horrors of my childhood, and I wasn't going to let history repeat itself.

Immediately upon hearing this news, I contacted the school. I was so sad that my daughter didn't tell me about the bullying sooner. The only topic Shaylee had vocalized prior to the counseling session was that she wanted me to stop writing the daily notes. She did not give me a reason why, and I never would have guessed it was because of cruel actions by classmates. What else goes on in my children's lives that I know nothing about?

There was only one week left in the school year, and her elementary school was busy with year-end events. There was a track and field day, a 'Fun Day' filled with games, and even a fourth-grade send-off with pizza and bowling. Shaylee didn't want to attend any of them. The family counselor wrote a note of permission to opt-out of those events since they weren't academic activities. I contacted the school, and they accepted the conditions. From there, I made an agreement with Shaylee: She had to finish the school year strongly by attending class each day, but she ONLY had to be there for the academic sessions – no more stressful celebrations with classmates. Fortunately, she honored our deal and successfully made it to the end of fourth grade.

After just two meetings with the family counselor, Shaylee had started opening up to me a lot more. She took the advice of 'letting emotions out' very seriously. The counselor had given Shaylee a journal to write and draw in, and it seemed to be helping her reflect. The counselor also reminded her that it was okay to talk about frustrating matters with trusted people. Shaylee went through a period of locking me in her room so that no one would interrupt. She would tell me all about her day. It was so comforting to see the spark in my daughter's eyes steadily return.

I asked Shaylee if she wanted to attend a private Christian school in fifth grade instead of staying in the same public school district, but she said she wanted to give it another try. I was proud of her perseverance and could see that Shaylee was ready to take on anything! That is until fifth grade began. Just two and a half weeks into the 2018 school year, her tears returned. After the third time of me walking Shaylee into the building and leaving her hyperventilating in the office, I'd had enough. The very next day, I enrolled Shaylee in the local Christian school. The atmosphere was incredibly loving, and we were welcomed with open arms. Tim and I never doubted our decision to switch schools or get her additional therapy. A bit of attention and reflection can be the most powerful tool when someone needs help. Shaylee has thrived in this smaller school, and I am so happy that we could make the proper adjustments for her needs.

 3 John 1:4 ~ I have no greater joy than to hear that my children are walking in the truth.

PUPPY POWER!

Sometimes you will never know the value of a moment
until it becomes a memory.

~ Theodor Seuss Geisel (Dr. Seuss)

A couple of months ago, I was invited to attend a Reiki Retreat near my hometown, approximately eight hours away. I desperately needed some time to recharge, but I wasn't sure how my family would deal with my few days of absence. Tim had to work out of town unexpectedly, and me leaving the kids with no one to take care of them felt wrong. It started looking like the only solution was for me to cancel my trip... sometimes, I get frustrated because it feels like I'm the only one making sacrifices. Plus, it was sad to abandon Brody and Holly on the weekend of their homecoming dance and leave Shaylee when she's feeling down. Everyone was pressuring me to stay home, and I was beginning to feel overwhelmed.

Suddenly, my phone rang. My close friend was on the other end of the line, and I couldn't help but express all of my concerns to her. I sobbed and sputtered out a meager explanation of why I couldn't leave my children for the weekend. She wasted no time on pity and told me to get my act together! My kids would be fine, and the grandparents could help. She even offered to accompany me on the eight-hour drive and weekend retreat. Her advice helped me regain some composure, and, with a sigh of relief, I took her up on the generous offer. After talking things through, everything seemed so much more doable. I guess I just needed someone to listen.

So, I asked my parents and mother-in-law if they would be willing to chip in. They were more than happy to watch over the kids until Tim returned home. I was so grateful that my friend called when she did – her support saved me! I definitely wouldn't have gone to this retreat without the help of her wisdom and patience.

Upon our arrival at the retreat on Friday afternoon (September 28), I knew God had meant for me to come here. One of the female leaders, in particular, turned out to be a true angel. When my friend and I approached the house, I recall this woman strolling outdoors and spreading around the smoke of burning incense. She was smudging, or energetically cleansing, around the home our group had rented for the getaway. She then asked all of us to stand on the porch so she could smudge us too! I was excited about all the good energy and enthusiastically stood in line. When it was my turn to get smudged, the woman grabbed my arm and pulled me aside. She mentioned that I had brought a lot of dead souls with me and went on to say that they were unintentionally drawing from my energy. I told her that I was recovering from a stem cell transplant and had lost quite a few friends to cancer.

At the time, I was still underweight and weak – so much so that it was noticeable to outsiders. She said that I needed to be careful at appointments located in the hospital because people die there, and their spirits follow light to get to heaven. The dead sometimes get confused and latch on to the bright lights of people, thinking that it will lead them to their eternal salvation. I wasn't angry with the lost souls, as I would probably want to follow the light too, but I needed to learn how to rid myself of them. Their attachment seemed to be preventing both of us from efficiently moving forward. I do not want my light to get drained.

The perceptive woman continued in her smudging of the house, and I stood there in awe for a moment, thinking, "What just happened?" Her words had come and gone quickly, but they made complete sense. I headed straight to my bedroom and jotted down notes of our brief encounter.

Just as I was rejoining the crowd of ladies, this same woman asked if there was someone named "Mary" in the group. I shyly raised my hand and uttered, "I'm Mary." She said, "Don't be frightened. I'm a medium, please come with me." She resumed her smudging ritual as we traveled upstairs in the three-story house.

The medium said that the spirit of a little boy was crying, and he refused to leave until he could speak with me. At first, I had no idea who this little boy could be. I reflected for a moment and asked the medium if the boy was a former student of mine who had passed away years ago. She shook her head. Then, all of a sudden, my hairdresser's son came to mind, and, again, I questioned if this was the child who wanted to speak with me. I shared that he had passed away after receiving a stem cell transplant and that complications prevented his relapse of acute myeloid leukemia from being cured.

Immediately following my inquiry, she began to sob and told me that the tears flowing down her face did not belong to her; they had come from the boy's energy flowing through her. She told me that he was hugging me at that moment, saying, "I love you so much! I want to let you know that you shouldn't feel bad or guilty because you survived and I didn't. I'm very happy now and not in any pain. I tried my best to make it through, but surviving was too hard for me. This was my first time on earth, and my contract was done." The medium continued in her translation by saying that I really needed to talk to his mom. My former hairdresser had many questions that only I could help answer, and she needs to speak with someone who's been through leukemia too – with someone who understands.

Through tears of my own, I apologized to him for being too scared to call his mom after I had heard about his death. I thought it would be too difficult for her to visit with me in this raw period of grief. I also told him that I did not know he had passed away until months later, and at that point, I wasn't sure what to do or say. He assured me that his mom would like to hear from me, and I agreed to contact her.

The boy wasn't finished speaking with me yet, though, and the medium continued to relay his messages. She said he was around my family often – especially Shaylee. I was astounded that the woman knew Shaylee's name – her knowledge only further confirmed that this boy's spirit was indeed here. He knew Shaylee was going through a difficult time at school and that she was seeing a therapist to help overcome anxiety. The boy went on to say that he knew Shaylee had been searching for dogs on my cell phone before school most mornings to help ease her nerves (we used this strategy for Shaylee to think about something she loved, such as dogs, instead of the long drive to school). In fact, she pleaded for our family to get another dog on a daily basis.

For this reason, he thought my family should get a miniature goldendoodle because he knew it would help us. Plus, this breed of dog has beautiful, golden curly hair, just as he did. My former hairdresser's son wanted to be remembered by us. The medium relayed his final message: "Promise me you will get one, and name it after me, whether it is male or female." He said Shaylee had already picked the puppy out when she was searching for dogs on the internet, but I didn't realize it.

Again, I could not believe how much he knew about us! His soul must have been around my family and me for quite a while. I had never met the medium before, so I have no clue how else she could have gotten this obscure information. When the boy-soul was ready to depart, he said he was going to hang out with Shaylee. I repeated my promise to connect with his mother and get a dog to name after him in reply. And as a final thought, I expressed my love for him and thanked him for reaching out to me. I know how difficult that must have been for him to do. Talking to this brave soul healed a wound I didn't even know I had.

Early Sunday morning, when the retreat was coming to an end, the medium, who was now a friend, wanted to visit with me privately. She pulled me into a separate room and pointed out that the time was 7:11 a.m. (this time will be significant in the next story). Our conversation was even more helpful to my healing process. She told me that I had briefly entered the spirit world when I was sick and had chosen to come back for my children. Tears rolled down my cheeks. She confirmed that I wasn't just imagining my 'breath of life' in the hospital in 2014. The woman went on to say, "You need to remember to step into your higher self. You are a divine mother with a bright light and lovely aura. Leukemia has packed its bags and is gone forever. The Divine contract of this illness is complete. There is no reason to fear its return. When your mind begins to spiral into negative thoughts, visualize a train stopped at a station in front of you. Shove all your fears into large bags and throw them onto the train. And once all of the bags are on board, watch the train depart, taking your baggage to God." This mental imagery has been very helpful in times when uncertainty revisits. Next, she handed me a pendulum to assist with Reiki treatments. Pendulums are divination tools used to help detect imbalances, or energy blocks, in the body (primarily at chakra points). I had never used one before, but I was eager to learn.

I left the retreat with nothing but gratitude and love for the medium and my other sisters. Over the weekend, we concentrated on utilizing Reiki energy to heal ourselves and others. Our group had opportunities to share reports of personal journeys, connecting experiences to each activity we undertook. The space felt safe, and I often participated in group discussions. After having survived CANcer, I've realized the importance of speaking up. Life is too short not to say what is on our minds. Of course, I still have my moments of insecurity, but I am proud of how far I've come.

This weekend, I learned that the deceased reap the rewards of healing energy as well. We sent Reiki energy to the land of devastation, cleansing it of war and destruction from the past. We also had discussions about the importance of affirmations and how the repetition of positive phrases helps accomplish goals. Affirmations can reduce stress, provide a stronger sense of self-worth, and help overcome negative thought patterns. I continue to remind myself that there are no permanent injuries. We can transform any bad habit by implementing a positive approach and practice.

When making affirmations, it's imperative to vocalize the statements as if they're already true – use "I am…" notation. For example, "I am joyful and courageous." It's best, at least for me, to vocalize these manifestations first thing in the morning. It's helpful to establish positivity from the get-go. I've posted affirmations on the refrigerator, on mirrors, in my car… honestly, anywhere I will notice them. While at the retreat, we wrote affirmations on colorful strips of paper for ourselves and each other. Each declaration was folded into the shape of a star and discreetly placed in personally-labeled jars. At the end of the retreat, each of us took the jar with our name on it. We could pluck a star of inspiration from the jar, open it, and read its kind message on any given day.

Our group also talked about visualizations – they can be super effective in redirecting our frame of mind. Utilizing imagery was a simple technique for me to master, especially during meditation. Here is an example from a chakra-clearing workshop: We visualized cutting energetic umbilical cords, chains, bonds, links, and hooks that could still be attached to our navel. The lines that not only kept us bound to our biological children but also our traumas, illnesses, fears, and concerns.

During this activity, tears streamed down my cheeks at the thought of pure freedom. I continue to practice this visualization periodically – environmental threats have the ability to latch on when we least expect them to. We also made prayer bundles for one of our last exercises, looping them through a roped chain that we could hang outdoors and burn.

Finally, I learned how to smudge, and we made smudge sticks (that we got to take home) to cleanse our house. I was told that we can ask our spirit guides or spiritual team to cleanse our homes for us too. Chanting the Ho'Oponopono (pronounced: HO – oh – Po-no – Po-no) Forgiveness Prayer during the cleanse was especially healing. The Ho'Oponopono mantra consists of four simple sentences that initiate the process of forgiveness, love, and harmony in troubled relationships. Its recitation permits freedom to 'cut' frayed connections and rectify severed relationships. The repetition of this prayer soothed my soul.

When I got home from this life-changing retreat and everyone was settled into bed at my house, I told Tim about what had happened with the medium and my former hairdresser's son.

He was very moved by the story and immediately agreed to purchase a miniature goldendoodle. The following morning, Tim and I took the two younger kids to school and then made a stop at the store. As we were leaving, I got a call from my chiropractor's office because I was late for my appointment (which I had completely forgotten about). Tim rushed me there and waited for me in the seating area by the receptionists' station.

While I was in the backroom, Tim overheard the receptionist visiting with another patient about her miniature goldendoodle and how much she loved her. Of course, Tim couldn't help himself and joined in on their conversation, getting the breeder's phone number right away. The receptionist said there was a six-to-eight-month waiting list. I decided to call the number anyway and left a message, hoping the breeder would call back soon. Tim and I discussed how different this morning would have been if I hadn't forgotten about my appointment. If I had been there on time, I would never have found out about the puppy. Hopefully, it was meant to be.

The breeder returned my call later that day and said she had *one* female puppy left. Apparently, another family had already claimed the puppy, but they found out that their apartment didn't allow pets. As a result, she said the other family had *just* canceled on the puppy over the weekend. It was even more 'meant to be' than we thought. Tim and I committed to purchasing the miniature goldendoodle before we even hung up the phone. The eight-week-old female puppy was ours. The kids were amazed by the magical story from my retreat and were even more thrilled that it meant we were getting a new puppy. I collected all the necessary puppy supplies and drove nearly two hours to pick up my sweet dog only a few days later!

Don't worry – I didn't forget about the other part of my promise. After picking up the goldendoodle, I decided to send a direct message on Facebook to my former hairdresser. Since I didn't have her phone number, I asked her to call me for important information. Several days passed before I received a response. She wrote that life was busy with her new baby boy, and it would be best to communicate through messenger with whatever I wanted to tell her. I was really torn about what to do after her semi-dismissive response. I didn't feel that the information about her son should be written in a message, so I decided it was best to discuss normal pleasantries instead.

Since my choice didn't necessarily honor the promise, I wanted to check in with my medium friend and ask for some advice. The wise woman promptly emailed me back and said that the little boy was with her at the moment. She said that he was so disappointed in his mom's response, and it was upsetting that she wouldn't open up to me. She assured me that he knew I did my best and said he released me from the promise. It was comforting to know it was okay to let go of my commitment. My former hairdresser's son said that he checks on his mother sometimes and that his baby brother can see him. This news made me very happy. In the email, my friend went on to say that I was no longer a survivor – I was a winner. She told me that I could visualize a healing bubble around his mother to aid in her recovery from grief.

In my initial email, I had also included the story of how I got our puppy and shared a cute photo. My medium friend told me that she loved the puppy, as it is *exactly* what she had seen in her mind's eye when the little boy showed her the dog at the retreat. My young friend (the little boy) thanked me for adopting the goldendoodle.

Our new furry companion is a real blessing to our family. She has really helped ease our dynamics. Strangely, I thought we got her to help Shaylee through challenging situations at school, but we've noticed our female friend has a strong bond with Tim. The pup is so loved, and we will always treasure the special way she came into our lives. She has since become a certified therapy dog and has opportunities to visit places all over the community, including schools, libraries, and nursing homes. Our dog is undoubtedly a reminder of that little boy, brightening up our lives with her golden-hazel eyes, sandy-blonde curly hair, and light brown nose.

 Isaiah 43:19 ~ See, I am doing a new thing! Now it springs up; do you not perceive it? I am making a way in the wilderness and streams in the wasteland.

THE SIGNIFICANCE OF GRAPES

Your peace is more important than driving yourself crazy trying to understand why something happened the way it did. Let it go.

~ Mandy Hale

Shortly after returning from the Reiki Retreat, I decided that we needed to have a family meeting. All of us gathered together in the living room and knew that we were about to have a very serious discussion. Just a few days prior, Holly had gotten extremely upset to the point of tears, and I felt that we all needed to talk about it. Here is some necessary background (keep in mind that there are two sides to every story, and this is my interpretation): A nearly-empty bowl of grapes was resting on the countertop, and Holly was trying to pack her lunch before school started. She became frustrated that there was no fresh fruit and vocalized that she feels I never listen when she asks for certain items from the store. She deemed the grapes "rotten" and unusable for her lunch, which stressed her out because now she wouldn't have a snack between school and her extracurricular activities. It was a simple problem, but it seemed to push her over the edge that day. I admit, I didn't handle her annoyance very well.

At that moment, I felt personally attacked and responded to her complaints by saying, "Seriously, I'm doing the best I can. Stop being so dramatic over grapes. I have enough going on right now and don't need your attitude piled on top of it!" Again, looking back, I realize how much of a mistake that response was. Holly replied, "It's not about the grapes, and it's *not* about *you*! Why do you always make *everything* about yourself?" And from there, she left the house for school. Ouch. This type of misunderstanding was starting to become a common occurrence between Holly and me. She and Tim get into spurts of disagreements as well, and I'm beginning to realize that we may not fully understand each other's points of view.

Looking back, I see that Holly had given up so much when I got sick. She sacrificed time with friends, time for rest, and time to just be a kid. From Holly's point of view, the *one* thing she had asked for was fresh grapes, and, although it was an honest mistake on my part, she had probably viewed it as her needs being dismissed yet again. I hadn't heard the real meaning behind her words.

After her outburst, Holly sent me a text **at 7:11 a.m.** while Brody was driving them to school. Let me tell you... what she had sent me caused some major alarm. In her text, Holly opened up to me about feelings of deep sadness and hopelessness. This information surprised me because her personality was typically so bright. She shared that she's happier at school than she is at home – school feels like the only place where she can be herself. Holly added that the second she walks through our door, she feels like she's met with constant invalidation and gaslighting, forcing her into defense mode. She ended the solemn message by saying she no longer had the energy left to explain herself or make any more justifications. No one ever listens, and she doesn't know what to do to make it stop.

Her text broke my heart. What had happened to our family? Where did my parenting theory of letting my kids speak their truths go? I feel that I've been so focused on my health and keeping everyone happy that I neglected to notice Holly's internal suffering. My job as a parent is to make her feel heard, and in the situation this morning, I failed.

I chose to respond to Holly's sad message with nothing but LOVE and thanked her for telling me how she felt. Additionally, when I noticed the time she had sent the text 7:11 a.m., I was immediately reminded of my conversation with the medium at the retreat. She had given me her phone number and said to call anytime, but I didn't think I would need to contact her this soon. I wanted to know if there was a reason she brought up the time (7:11 a.m.) during our visit that Sunday morning. Perhaps she had more wisdom to share to help me through this challenging situation.

After dropping the youngest two kids off at school, I decided to call the medium and leave a voicemail. Fortunately, she called me back promptly. The woman was so helpful and thought it would be beneficial for me to visit with another sister from the retreat (a retired licensed counselor) about what had happened with Holly. I thanked her for the suggestion and immediately connected with the former counselor. She suggested that I give Holly time to tell me how she felt without having to fear a negative response from me. I needed to make her feel heard and appreciated, as that is not a sentiment Holly thought she'd been shown lately. This new sisterhood was just what I needed, and I am blessed to be part of the strong group retreat attendees. I expressed immense gratitude to my sister and planned to speak with Holly when she got out of school.

After picking her up, Holly and I had a gentle conversation with no yelling and no anger. She cried, and I actively listened to what had been plaguing her, apologizing for not being more attentive. I received many hugs from Holly that evening, and she seemed relieved to have let go of the emotional baggage. I also spoke with Tim and the other children to be more mindful of each other's feelings. We need to think before we speak. Our home felt calmer and more peaceful after that night.

With these recent realizations, I began to understand that most, if not all of us, have underlying feelings of worry. For some unknown reason, we hold onto those silent fears and let them consume us until we reach a breaking point. I was not going to let those intrusive thoughts latch on to my family or me any longer. Each of us needs to feel free enough to release our burdens.

During the family meeting I had scheduled, I explained that we were all living in F.E.A.R. (False Evidence Appearing Real). And I think that a lot of this was coming from my CANcer struggles. I explained that "fear" is what causes problems – the threatening thing itself is not to blame for our concerns. We each had taken on roles to help our family move forward when I was sick, and I recognize that those sacrifices are difficult to compensate for. But, fundamentally, family takes care of family, and that's what we did. I told my kids that I was very proud of them for stepping up to help when we needed it most. Tim and I assured them that, from now on, we would honor *all* thoughts and feelings – no matter how bizarre they may initially seem. We all have personal viewpoints related to our experiences, after all. I even held a wand with a glowing star at the tip to remind us of light and love. I explained that whoever holds the wand has the power to speak their truth, uninterrupted. We passed it around as many times as needed so that each person could release their afflictions.

If they didn't feel like sharing their feelings just yet, that was okay too. We can always take our sorrows to Jesus. What's important is that, from now on, we are no longer going to try to suppress our pain. Holly's rotten grapes meant so much more than I had assumed, and I urge everyone to look deeper into your interactions. Stop and think before snapping at someone unnecessarily. Above all, strive to respond with love.

 Ephesians 4:16 ~ He makes the whole body fit together perfectly. As each part does its own special work, it helps the other parts grow, so that the whole body is healthy and

growing and full of love.

Tangible Blessings

Prayer flags have been an interest of mine from the moment I first saw them at my kayaking retreat in 2015. Back then, I was so inspired that when I returned home, I immediately researched the meaning behind them to learn more. However, as the days turned into months and the months into years, I became busy with other life happenings and forgot about making my own prayer flag.

Since then, I've experienced a sweat lodge and a Reiki Retreat with tobacco prayer bundles. These indulgences reminded me of my former interest in the flags and reestablished my passion. Although prayer flags and prayer bundles have the same purposes, they look nothing alike; the main difference is that by wrapping the prayer in a bundle, with or without tobacco, you *capture* the prayer, and the flags are simply pieces of fabric that carry the prayer out into the wind. Tobacco has traditionally been used by the eastern nations, including Cherokee, Lakota, and Cree – it's considered their most sacred and cherished medicinal plant. When burned, tobacco is believed to be a gift for the Great Spirit or Creator in exchange for blessings.

Our Reiki group took a unique approach to making our tobacco prayer bundles, which was perfect because there is no set way to make them. Solid square-shaped pieces of assorted-colored fabric were laying on a table. Each color represented a category and was labeled accordingly. For example, the white cloth symbolized a prayer for healing, red for ancestors, yellow for giving thanks, and so on. Strips of paper were provided to write a prayer, name, phrase, or word of things needing to be released or received. The paper is then folded and placed within the chosen colored cloth alongside Native American tobacco. The four corners of the fabric were cinched by looping a string around the bundle, forming a long chain.

When I began this exercise, I thought of all my loved ones. I added each of their names to a piece of paper and meticulously wrapped them in the cloths of my prayer chain. However, when it came to thinking of my personal intentions, it was hard for me to come up with anything other than releasing leukemia. It was crazy to me that I just sat in silence with total emptiness in my mind. Why did cancer always creep its way into my thoughts? Maybe it was because I wanted to live a free life more than anything else.

I glanced around the room and actively listened to the group of ladies, hoping that their sporadic chatting would spark some new ideas of my own. I ended up writing down a couple more things before moving on to the next activity, but I still didn't feel like my chain was complete. Fortunately, the materials were left out on the table for the rest of the weekend, just in case anyone wanted to return to it during free time.

The following morning, creative ideas for a prosperous, joyful life flowed out of me; I made another tobacco prayer chain, this time with ease. Perhaps I just needed time to process what it was that I actually desired? I generally put the needs of others before my own, as most mothers do, so this internal shift of priorities brought me back to the freedom of my childhood. I was eager to see how *my* desires would unfold.

When I returned home with my two chains of tobacco prayer ties, I draped them across my desk for nearly a year. I'm not sure why I didn't hang them outdoors or even burn them right away as some did at the retreat, but I guess there was no set rule of that either. I just did what felt right to me. Then, one day out of the blue, I noticed the colorful prayer bundles and decided it was finally time to burn them. I went outside and privately had a ceremony of flames. First, I set my intention. Then, I gently placed the prayer ties in an empty stewpot and lit them on fire. I symbolically released my requests through the smoke rising to the heavens. Their destruction revitalized my hope. I could feel God's celestial smile when he received my messages.

 Psalm 20:5 ~ May we shout for joy over your victory and lift up our banners in the name of our God. May the Lord grant all your requests.

EIGHT

A NEW AWARENESS

Life is anything but stable. As humans, it's easy to get stuck going through the motions… but think about how much you grow from trudging through mud and how invigorating it feels to soar through the air. This *instability* is the key to becoming the best version of yourself. Risk is scary, but with the trust of God, leaps of faith are always worthwhile. I cannot wait to share my new awareness with you, and I pray that you experience some gambles of your own. A life with meaning is a life worth living.

PURPOSEFUL DRIVEN FORCE

Yesterday I was clever, so I wanted to change the world.
Today I am wise, so I am changing myself.

~ Rumi

After undergoing the stem cell transplant and surpassing two near-death experiences, I am very in tune with my body. I've had a growing awareness that I haven't been taking care of my personal needs for some time, and I now realize the importance of putting my own oxygen mask on first. I think that the best place to start in this self-care process is pursuing my interests.

I wanted to continue learning more about Reiki and gaining confidence in universal energy. I wasn't sure if I should retake Level Two since I hadn't practiced it in a while or just move onto Level Three. After giving it some thought, I signed up for the Reiki Two course again. Joining the class a second time was a wise choice for me. It had been nearly two years since taking it with the prior Reiki Master/Teacher, and I didn't use it enough throughout that time to fully comprehend the material. This time around, I was primarily focused on the concept of "Release the need to understand." This idea was a struggle for me to accept, as my personality type needs to know why and how before making sense of things. Additionally, energy is confusing in itself – universal energy just knows where to go for maximum healing.

When the Reiki Two class began in early March 2019, I was glad to be in a small group. We had several opportunities to practice energy sessions on each other while our teacher supervised from a distance. The instructor himself also worked on each of us briefly near the end of the course. Being in a Reiki class with other people was a whole new experience.

During my session with our teacher, I felt very relaxed, and I closed my eyes with an intention for the highest good. He asked if I came from a strict family. I wasn't sure how to respond. I told him that I was at peace with my upbringing, and it was a loving environment, for the most part. He went on to say that I still feel the need to prove myself and asked me to picture a strong, empathetic, and compassionate person. Immediately, I blurted out, "Wonder Woman!" He chuckled in agreement. At that moment, my eyebrows shook and twitched uncontrollably. I saw sparkling lights resembling the brightness of scattered stars underneath my closed eyelids. My teacher continued saying that I had a big goal in the future, and it would be like a birth from the womb. I asked him if it was my book. He didn't know exactly what it meant, but it could mean that it would be about **nine months** – likeness to a pregnancy. Regardless, he said to imagine myself as Wonder Woman when I need to reach a creative state of mind.

When our time together came to a close, the Reiki Master/Teacher performed the Level Two attunement ceremony. During the event, he had a few personal words for each of us. He told me that he sees the color purple in my aura (the highest vibrational frequency – close connection with the Spirit Realm and life energy) with a large mountain behind me.

At the end of that same month, I took Reiki Level Three with the same Reiki Master/Teacher. It was everything that I thought it would be and then some! Like before, participants practiced new techniques by working on each other. Reiki Level Three concluded with another attunement ceremony, and once again, my instructor shared a few words for each of us. His closing words to me were:

> *"You are a healer and always have been; maybe now you're recognizing it. It might have been passed down from ancestors, possibly a female. Don't let illness get in your way. You knew you would overcome and beat it with God by your side. You healed yourself in this way. Your family is getting more used to the idea of Reiki. It is not something they understand, but they are growing to accept this part of your life. You are a healer and a Teacher, with a capital 'T.' I don't know exactly what that means, but time will tell. Perhaps it's in the field of teaching students in another capacity? Reiki energy emanates off you."*

Both ceremonies were blissful, and I was so grateful for his confirmation that I was on the right path. I cannot wait to see what is to come.

BURNING CELEBRATION

Sometimes you get the best light from a burning bridge.

~ Don Henley

My high school classmate from so many years ago and I made plans to take our kids to the Henry Doorly Zoo on June 21. It was such a gorgeous day. Colby and Shaylee were able to tag along, but Brody and Holly had other plans, and Tim was working out of town. It had been years since I had been to the zoo with any of my children.

After a long day of walking to see all the animals, we arrived at the Children's Adventure Trails. The kids were free to roam and climb the equipment. It was a magical place, full of wonder. Their temporary distraction with the playground gave my friend and me time to visit about how life had been since the stem cell transplant. I told her of my previous desire to have a burning ceremony on day one hundred, detailing my failure to accomplish that goal. She said, "You should do it today, on the Summer Solstice!" I immediately replied, "What a great idea!" I decided to have the burning ceremony on this lengthy, warm day to make the end of my journey feel special.

When we arrived home, I rushed to my closet and grabbed the dreaded CANcer box. Motivation was on my side, and I was ready to finally follow through with my intentions. Inside, years of items rested in battered piles, and I quickly sorted through the ones to be discarded. Colby and Shaylee helped me carry all the papers and unwanted reminders to the burn barrel near our shop. We loaded it to the top and lit it with a torch. The 'burning' ceremony featured all the items in my CANcer box that no longer served me. It was such a great release to see everything erupt into flames. The destruction made my victory over cancer feel real, but I realized it would not change the road I've traveled or erase memories. CANcer is a part of my identity now; I'm simply not going to let it define me. I am healed. The kids took a couple of pictures and videos of me tossing my hair clippings into the flames and praising God for granting me life. Colby, Shaylee, and I had a great time, and I wouldn't have changed any moment of it.

I recommend this multisensory approach to anyone struggling to let go of burdens. If you don't have physical items to burn, write a note or a letter about the situation as another option. You could also have a simple conversation with God and ask Him to cleanse you from all encumbrances. There is a lot of power in removing unwanted memories, thoughts, and items. I know this from experience. I leave you with this quote by Amit Ray, "Everyone has the fire, but the champions know when to ignite the spark."

 Romans 15:13 ~ May the God of hope fill you with all joy and peace as you trust in him, so that you may overflow with hope by the power of the Holy Spirit.

MAKE IT COUNT

Sometimes you will never know the value of a moment until it becomes a memory.

~ Theodor Suess Geisel (Dr. Seuss)

Some moments in our life are so vivid that they stick with us for a lifetime. Moments such as these can invoke lingering sadness, spiraling excitement, or enlightening lessons. Regardless of the result, their messages are impossible to ignore. Here is a description of one of these rare instances from my childhood:

I remember this occasion like it was yesterday. My aunt took my cousins and me shopping when I was in my early teens. Just as we walked into a department store, I noticed a stand of lip gloss tubes filled with every color imaginable. Immediately, I set forth to find the ideal tint for me. Alas, I found the perfect one! After purchasing a shade of soft pink shimmering shell gloss, I told myself that I would take excellent care of it. I bought it with my own money and had always valued my possessions. I think this trait of understanding worth comes from my parents. They often told my brother and me, "Some people don't have anything except for the shirts on their backs. So, you should be grateful for everything you have." I took their message seriously in all circumstances and vowed to never mistreat my lip gloss.

When I arrived home, I took the tube out of its package and placed it in my makeup bag. Frequently, I grabbed the lip gloss and stared at its smooth consistency, admiring the beauty and quality. Even with this admiration, however, not once did I dare to actually apply the precious sheen to my lips. Don't get me wrong, I knew it would look lovely on me, and I desperately wanted to put it to use, but the thought of preserving its beauty was far more comforting. I felt that if I were to use this lip gloss, it would eventually be gone, and I wouldn't have my valuable item anymore. I needed to take care of my possessions, and so, in keeping with this frame of mind, I waited for the perfect time to apply it to my lips. As time went by, the tube remained in its stale location.

Sometimes my friends and I would get together to put on our makeup before heading out for an evening of fun. It was always entertaining to update each other on the latest news and anticipate how our adventurous night would pan out – especially if there were boys involved! On one particular occasion, my friend grabbed the lip gloss from my makeup bag and started marveling over it. She quickly opened the tube and spread the gloss over her lips. She said the color was amazing and looked perfect on her. I couldn't believe my eyes! I had kept this lip gloss so safe and untainted until that moment. Unfortunately, I was stern with my friend and asked her to check with me before using my makeup. I was so disappointed that the seal had been broken – especially since I wasn't even the first one who got to use it. In that moment, it felt that all my efforts had been for nothing. This entire situation seems so silly, right?

I often put so much value on even the smallest items that I didn't allow myself to enjoy them. For instance, when I was in my late teens, another aunt gifted me her elegant ring, studded with a large pearl and three small diamonds. This exquisite ring held sentimental value to her, and she had owned it since childhood. Since my aunt only had boys, she wanted to pass it on to me, and it meant the world that she trusted me to take care of something so important. Do I still have the ring? Yes, but sadly, it still sits in the original box, never worn and unscathed. I was too afraid that I would damage it or lose a diamond. My ring looks as brilliant as the day I received it, and I've fulfilled my promise to watch over it.

Regrettably, leaving it in that case for all these years seems to have made it lose the luster that a ring should have. It's about time I wore this precious gift while I still have time to appreciate it. As for the lip gloss? It ended up in the trash, unused by me, except for a special occasion or two. It became old and expired, lacking its former smooth texture and shine.

I learned a lesson when I threw my favorite lip gloss in the trash: Don't let the things you love go to waste just because you're afraid of ruining them. Cherishing possessions is different than admiring them from afar or locking them away; if we hold onto things too tightly, they will lose their worth. So, go ahead and put on the lip gloss! Wear the ring! Enjoy all that life offers.

 Ecclesiastes 3:12-13 ~ So I concluded there is nothing better than to be happy and enjoy ourselves as long as we can. And people should eat and drink and enjoy the fruits of their labor, for these are gifts from God.

Repeat, Recharge

In July, I had the opportunity to join some of my fellow Reiki sisters in a Level Three Reiki class taught by three instructors near my hometown in western Nebraska. I talked to Tim about it, hoping he would support my decision to retake this Reiki level because, of course, it was an additional expense. I believed this would be a great review and solidify my newfound confidence in energy work. Tim gave me his blessing, and I anxiously read more books to fit as much knowledge in before class began.

The first day of class was mind-blowing, and I knew that I was meant to be there. Each teacher had unique qualities and experiences that enlightened us in different ways. When I arrived at class on the second day, I told them about the vision I woke up to that morning: Files were being downloaded into my mind, and from a newfound perspective of clarity, I saw myself stepping into my higher self, with both feet in, through faith.

Later that day, I volunteered to lay on a massage table while the teacher demonstrated a technique to the class. Afterward, she told me of *her* vision – she said I stepped into my higher self with both feet in, and I had gold Wonder Woman boots on. Upon hearing this, tears streamed down my cheeks. I was astonished! She didn't even know about my Wonder Woman connection! It further confirmed the significance of the interaction with my former Reiki instructor. When I shared this revelation with the group, they cheered alongside me, happy that I felt confident in my identity.

Since evolving my awareness, I've learned to be more gentle and kind to myself. I cannot let F.E.A.R. (False Evidence Appearing Real) and doubt take control of situations in my life. I've found that my inner being is equipped with the tools to overcome whatever is in my path.

As I continue on my healing journey, I feel as if I am generating a rebirth and expansion of myself. By letting go of anxiety, I am permitting myself to create space for the tasks I love. Sometimes we must step into sovereignty and embrace randomness. Guidance, while often unclear, will sporadically point us to our destiny. Plus, life would be boring if it were a straight line. I'm ready for all the twists and turns to come.

 Galatians 5:22 ~ But the fruit of the Spirit is love, joy, peace, patience, kindness, goodness, faithfulness, gentleness, self-control; against such things there is no law.

FINDING THE WORDS

Words are the most powerful thing in the universe…
Words are containers. They contain faith, or fear,
and they produce after their kind.

~ Charles Capps

Words are so powerful. Even the most basic forms of language can relay lasting messages – they reveal the meaning behind actions. And when words are pieced together to form sentences, they add another stroke of color to our miraculous painting of life. Words showcase all kinds of profound interpretations, ranging from building us up to breaking us down. Nonetheless, regardless of the tone of their impressions, words are difficult to overlook. Psalm 52:2 states, "The tongue devises mischiefs; like a sharp razor, working deceitfully."

The old saying, "Sticks and stones can break my bones, but words will never hurt me," is a sham. Spoken insults are so potent that their effects may be lifelong. Proverbs 12:18 states, "The words of the reckless pierce like swords, but the tongue of the wise brings healing." This piece of wisdom tells us to consider our choice of words before we speak, as our communication will determine how our relationships develop.

Now that I think about it, tongues may be the most difficult thing to control in our lives. Keep in mind that we, as humans, naturally speak thousands of words a day. It's only expected that a few tainted phrases will slip out. While most of these misspeaks are negligible, some will leave us with years of regret. Fortunately, we have the Word of the Bible to call upon for strength and guidance. God helps us realize that words are just as good at helping us apologize as they are at helping us hurt each other. Our outlook is what matters. (Fun fact: Women average 20,000 words a day and Men, only 7,000).

The reason words have been so intriguing to me lately is that August 22, 2019, marked two years since my stem cell transplant. I had a routine checkup with my oncologist a few weeks ago and was eager to fill out the *Post-Transplant Consent Form to Release Personal Information* from *Be The Match*. The form was submitted by my case manager, and I anxiously awaited a reply. My donor had the choice to either give me his personal information or decline. And no matter what he decided to do, it made me so happy that he would know I am alive and well – all thanks to the goodness of his heart – not to mention God and the excellent medical care team.

Back to the power of words, I am having a rough time figuring out what to say to the generous man who saved my life. What words can adequately express my gratitude? I've been waiting so long for the moment I could contact him, but now that it's here, I'm speechless. Proverbs 20:15 states, "Gold there is, and rubies in abundance, but lips that speak knowledge are a rare jewel."

On occasion, my friends may have heard me joke about my donor being muscular, tall, and handsome (with a full head of hair!) because it was *his* stem cells that gave me new DNA. I've imagined him possibly resembling the muscular German hunk from butter commercials, with his long golden locks and beefy stature, biting into an appealing morsel of goodness. On a serious note, no matter what he looks like, my donor will always be perfect in my eyes. His selflessness outweighs all.

In mid-September 2019, our faithful Lord showed favor upon my request to connect with my donor, and his contact information from *Be The Match* arrived in an email from my case manager at Nebraska Medicine. The subject line read "MR Donor Information Exchange." I paused for a minute, looked up to heaven, and smiled at God with appreciation. It took no time to read through the consent record and personal information. My donor provided me with his name, home address, phone number, email, and date of birth. All this time, I've been referring to him with a made-up name and image – now it was the moment of truth. His real name is Stephan... "Ahh, such a sophisticated, proper, well-rounded name," I thought. And he is from Germany, just as I had been told. I stopped for a moment, wondering what to do now. I wanted to take some time to think about the next steps before impulsively seeking him out (as if two years wasn't long enough).

I decided that each member of my family (Tim and the kids) would write a short paragraph about Stephan's impact on our lives. I wanted him to know how much his donation helped us all. Once finished, I'll send the writings with a personal letter of my own, along with some photos of us.

Back to the two-year post-transplant checkup, my day began with labs. Following those routine tests, I got a bone density screening and then went to the actual doctor's appointment. For some reason, I didn't feel as anxious about my test results this time around. I guess that sometime in the past five years of dealing with these appointments, I've realized that no matter how I feel, the results will not change. My blood work is independent from my emotions, and although a positive mindset is helpful, it can only go so far. That doesn't matter, though. At this stage in my journey, I'm genuinely joyful and literally feeling bursts of happiness in my soul. And to be honest, I don't recall the last time I really felt this way. I'm not saying I wasn't happy before, but rather that I am actually feeling my suffering disappear. The only way we can reach the core of our essence is to peel back the layers of burdens that block it from sight.

These blockages can be difficult to face, but we can't grow if we aren't willing to surrender our protective mechanisms. It helps to talk things out or write them down. There are so many relevant words in our vocabulary. Which ones are you going to use today? Perhaps no words are necessary at all – sometimes just a smile will do.

Proverbs 15:4 ~ The soothing tongue is a tree of life, but a perverse tongue crushes the spirit.

Letters to Stephan

Below are messages that my four children, husband, and I wrote to my stem cell transplant donor. It took several months to complete this task. Regardless, I emailed Stephan our letters on May 8, 2020. I hope he enjoys reading them and knows the positive impact he made in our lives.

Dear Stephan,

My name is Mary Robinson, and you graciously donated your life-giving stem cells nearly three years ago so that I may live. I can't believe it has taken me so long to write to you. It has been difficult for me to find adequate words to say, "Thank you." A while back, I wrote a passage on my CaringBridge site called *Finding the Words*. I am sharing portions with you because it expresses my gratitude in narrative form (I included those excerpts in my stories above). My letter ended with this:

At my two-year checkup, my doctor told me I was doing well. I asked, "Does this mean that I'M CURED?" And he said, "YES, I believe it does (with a smile). Just make sure to keep the stress level to a minimum." I have been waiting so long to hear those words. I will continue to have routine checkups and am so grateful to be alive and well. Thank you, Stephan, for saving my life – sending all my love.

With sincerest gratitude,

Mary Robinson

Dear Stephan,

I would like to introduce myself. My name is Tim Robinson. I am 48 years old and the father of four incredible children (Brody-19, Holly-17, Colby-14, and Shaylee-12). I am also the husband of the most wonderful woman I have ever known (Mary Jane Robinson-43). We have been married for twenty years and live in Fremont, Nebraska.

I am writing to thank you from the bottom of my heart for the gift of life that you gave not only to my wife, but to our entire family. We are people of faith and hold the Lord close to our hearts. You are someone we've never met (not yet anyway), and you returned my wife and my children's mother back to us! I cannot express the gratitude that I have for you. You are a very special individual to give your stem cells to a complete stranger.

I want you to know that my beautiful wife is here today, being the most wonderful mother to our four children and spreading her love and joy to everyone she meets because of your incredible gift, and of course, God! You are truly an inspiration. May God bless you and your family. I look forward to thanking you in person someday.

Sincerely,

Timothy Robinson

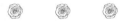

Dear Stephan,

Thank you so much for keeping my mom here on Earth, alive and well. I was willing to do what you did for my mom, but she had antibodies that would have rejected my stem cells, so I wasn't able to donate them. When we found that out, I didn't know what to do. I thought it was all over, but then *Be The Match* found you, and you were willing to save my mom – my mom – a complete stranger to you, and you did it anyway. I don't even know where to begin, except to say, "Thank you!" My mom is everything to me.

I am graduating high school this year, just living life to the fullest. I finished the football and wrestling seasons. Track practice was supposed to start, but we are all out of school because of the coronavirus. I completed all my requirements to graduate, though, and I am going to be a land surveyor. So glad my mom is here for our family.

Wish me luck!

Brody – 19 years old

Stephan,

I like to consider my life a patch of dirt filled with various assortments of plants. My siblings pose as cacti, prickly and menacing in most cases, but refreshing once you cut inside; my grandparents are willow trees, swaying slowly and calmly, seeping knowledge and wisdom; my dad is an obvious palm tree - he likes to relax and have fun; my mother, however, is much more difficult to pin down. You see, she is beautiful and nurturing – a flower, perhaps? But no, that's not right because she is also forgiving, determined, sophisticated, quirky, and full of advice. My mom is not someone who can be easily stepped on. I view her as the essence of life. She chooses to build me up, even when her own foundation is unsteady. Her selfless nature and unwillingness to accept unsatisfactory effort are what make her my role model. Without her guidance, I would be lost and confused. My mother is a tall pillar of hope and strength, which can be symbolized by none other than a *redwood tree*! It is thanks to you and God that her tree is still standing. The gift of my mother is more than I could ever ask for or deserve, and there is nothing I can do to repay the immense debt I owe you. I can't possibly voice how much I appreciate your donation. Thank you. Or, as you probably say it, Danke.

Holly – 17 years old

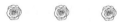

Dear Stephan,

Thank you for giving your stem cells to my mom. It takes a really good person to do that. Your donation really helped my family make it through this hard time. We don't know what we would've done if you wouldn't have donated.

Thank you,

Colby – 14 years old

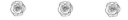

Dear Stephan,

Thank you for saving my mom. It means a lot to my family and me. Without you, my mom wouldn't be here, and we would all be in a very dark place. It takes a good heart and bright personality to do something like that. So, thank you!

Shaylee – 12 years old

 Proverbs 16:24 ~ Gracious words are a honeycomb, sweet to the soul and healing to the bones.

A HEALING TOUCH

Healing comes from taking responsibility: to realize that it is you
– and no one else – that creates your thoughts,
your feelings, and your actions.

~ Peter Shephard

Rewind to December 2019, I was skimming through one of my journaling notebooks to reflect on my writings. Suddenly, a small piece of torn paper fell out of the booklet and landed on my lap. It happened to be the contact information for a local Healing Touch group. Healing Touch is another universal energy therapy modality. The small piece of paper was given to me when I attended Reiki Two class about nine months ago. I set it down and told myself I would give the course some thought. A couple more days passed, and I couldn't stop thinking about Healing Touch, so I decided to make the call. The lady who answered directed me to the coordinator. I immediately phoned her and left a message. Shortly after, the coordinator returned my call, and we ended up visiting for a long time. It was as if we had known each other for years. I felt like I belonged in this community of healers, so I accepted her invitation to try a session with her. I was grateful for a chance to try it out before officially signing up for the first course.

The monthly healing touch practice group met the following week, and I discovered that it perfectly complemented my Reiki work! I felt so relaxed when I left that I immediately signed up for the upcoming class scheduled for February 2020. In the meantime, I was invited to attend their Healing Touch Open House and Workshop in January 2020. I didn't know what to expect or who would be there, but my intuition told me to go. It was more than I could have ever imagined! A woman presented us with a showcase of various medicinal herbs and tools used by shamans. Having lived with shamans for nearly two years, she shared learnings from their way of life and ancient healing techniques.

After the presentation, she offered Shamanic Healing Touch sessions with no charge, aside from a freewill donation. I eagerly scheduled a session with her that afternoon. Upstairs was an inviting space prepared for healing. A massage table stood in the center of the room, and the aroma of burning smudge wafted about. Toward the end of my session, she spoke in tongues. It was very peaceful. And when it came to a complete close, she told me:

> *"Keep writing – especially when it flows. And continue to write until it stops. Write about faith and manifestation – You manifested your outcome and kept your faith during health battles. Angels really like you and want to work with you. Keep trying to hear them. They want you to hear them – meditate on this. You may need to talk through feelings and emotional patterns with someone trusted in order to discover a new approach to let go of unwanted actions that do not serve you. Don't be afraid of the stigma surrounding that form of treatment. We all need healing from one thing or another."*

I was so grateful for her guidance because it confirmed my intuition regarding the supernatural occurrences in my life. Now I know that angels, spirit guides, and spirit animals are present whenever my lips tingle or a cool breeze brushes across my face with no explanation.

Energy follows thought, so we need to be conscious of what we say and think. Energy also moves with breath. By developing a creative state of mind, images of successful outcomes become much clearer. The stronger I believe in my goals, the more I can allow manifestation to flow directly in my favor. Frequently, I use affirmations to remind myself that I am strong, worthy, focused, and destined to continue learning about energy healing. I have a purpose.

John 14:12 ~ "Very truly I tell you, whoever believes in me will do the works I have been doing, and they will do even greater things than these, because I am going to the Father."

LIFE IS A DANCE – YOU LEARN AS YOU GO

You have the power to heal yourself, and you need to know that.
We think so often that we are helpless, but we're not.
We always have the power of our minds.
Claim and consciously use your power.

~ Louise Hay

February finally arrived, and I was prepared for the first Healing Touch class to begin. The course was outstanding! I learned so much more about energy work and how we can help others in their overall health. The client has control over their own healing, and the practitioner's job is to be the conduit for the release and acceptance of energy. In each of our sufferings, we come to know the truth about ourselves from the lessons we learn. Clearing energetic congestion allows us to reclaim our power, truth, and authentic self.

I love the idea of the client being in charge of their journey to good health and hadn't thought of it that way before. Being on the other side of healing has helped me realize just how much the process is dependent on the client. I also enjoy helping people reach their highest selves. When I engage with clients on their healing journey, I am simply raising their vibrational level to boost their body's recovery. This practice is what I am meant to do, so I decided to take all five courses. After completing the courses, I will do all the necessary work to become certified.

The second class was scheduled for the end of May 2020, and it couldn't have come fast enough. Healing Touch became my passion. In the meantime, I practiced my learnings from the previous class with my family. By this time, my family had started to open up to the idea of universal energy. They welcomed sessions with me and were more than willing to help me practice what I learned. Perhaps this willingness was because they began noticing positive changes in themselves after our sessions.

May arrived, and my confidence grew exponentially, especially as we learned new techniques and practiced with each other. I came to the realization that Healing Touch is the 'peace that passes all understanding' and acknowledged the ideas of:

1. Make no comparisons.

As humans, this isn't always easy to do. It reminds me of the quote, "Don't compare your life to others. There's no comparison between the sun and the moon. They shine when it's their time." Sometimes we get so caught up worrying about the talents of others that we lose sight of our own.

2. Make no judgments.

When we name deep-rooted actions that have been previously suppressed, those concerns lose their power over us. This strategy makes it much easier to release negativity. As clients tell their stories, practitioners must have unconditional positive respect. We don't know what life is like for someone else and might not know enough about their background to fully understand their circumstances, so what right do we have to judge them for their actions?

3. Delete the need to understand.

We may never know exactly how energy functions, but it seems to know just where to go and what to do. Why waste your time questioning it when energy is doing what is necessary for our prosperity?

After taking courses one and two, I came to understand how incredibly powerful touch is! When using Reiki, my hands had never touched the client's body, just floated above – not that touching wasn't an option, but it wasn't necessary for me. Besides, I didn't have a license to touch. The techniques were still doing their job. Of course, applying Reiki techniques without touch still yields great value, but as I learned more, I personally found even more value in *physical* contact. I wanted to be able to 'legally' place my hands on clients for whatever healing purposes they need. So, I was moved to become ordained. In the state of Nebraska, a license to touch is acknowledged if you are a doctor, nurse, certified nursing assistant, massage therapist, or ordained minister.

I met a retired teacher in our Healing Touch community who became ordained years ago for *her* license to touch. I asked her what organization she had gone through to complete the process, and she happily assisted me. I completed all the necessary forms and guidelines, and this retired teacher, who is now a dear friend, offered to perform my ordination ceremony personally. I gladly accepted. On Labor Day, September 7, 2020, we met at her house.

At the end of the ceremony, I lit a white tea candle placed in a green crystal candle holder. Right away, the white color of the candle reminded me of the crown chakra (spiritual) that starts with purple and transitions to white. The green color of the holder reminded me of the heart chakra (unconditional love). These colors were the perfect representation and symbolization of what was happening at that moment – committing to love and light with my whole heart.

Afterward, she took me on a shamanic spiritual animal journey to discover my spirit animal(s). I relaxed on a massage table, with my eyes closed, as she read a guided meditation that took me on a naturistic excursion. I envisioned a lush forest and began to wander through it. A couple of deer were in my peripheral, standing like statues, staring at me as they ate from the ground. A hawk flew above me, then drifted ahead. As I continued through the forest, it opened to a vast prairie. There was a tall cliff-like hill with a narrow waterfall on the other side, and the same hawk gracefully flew overhead again, landing on a shrub. I decided to sit by a nearby creek and scan the prairie.

From there, I began to notice something move toward me in the distance. As the image drew closer, I recognized a big mane around the animal's face and knew it had to be a lion. The lion approached with confidence and sat right next to me! A slight nudge from his nose signaled that it was okay for me to stroke his mane. We rested there peacefully for a bit. After a few moments, I decided to grasp the lion's thick fur and climb on top of him. I held on tightly as the lion stood up and dashed across the prairie. The wind pressed against us, and my hair unfurled behind me. A herd of deer parted ways for us to glide through them with ease, and as I looked into the sky, the same hawk was flying near us.

As much as I wanted to stay in this meditational state of joyful awareness, it was time for me to return to reality. The lion must have sensed this, and he returned me to the edge of the prairie. When I dismounted from the lion, he walked with me until it was time for him to stop. As I departed back to the real world, I turned around one last time and saw him sitting there, staring at me with love and trust. When I opened my eyes, I did nothing but lay there with amazement. Spiritual goosebumps were all over my body as I shared this mental adventure with my friend. I know my spirit animals are with me, ready to help any time.

Later that month, my official certificate of ordination came in the mail. I was overjoyed with the title: Reverend Mary Jane Robinson. I take pride in how far I have come, and that day, I made a promise to God that I would use this position to help people heal. Nothing eases pain and suffering like human touch.

 Proverbs 3:5-6 ~ Trust in the Lord with all your heart and lean not on your own understanding; in all your ways submit to him, and he will make your paths straight.

LOOK WITH A CHILD-LIKE CURIOSITY

If we experienced life through the eyes of a child,
everything would be magical and extraordinary.
Let our curiosity, adventure and wonder of life never end.

~ Akiane Kramarik

A couple of weeks after being ordained, it was time for me to start the third Healing Touch course. This class gave us time to experience the roles of a practitioner, a client, and an observer. It was a great way to put the positions of others into perspective. From there, we were asked to look through the lens of a child and be curious. What do you see, hear, smell, feel, and taste? It made me think of the movie *Hook* and Peter Pan's famous quote, "Come with me where dreams are born, and time is never planned." Peter Pan loved the make-believe games they played in Never Never Land. He never lost his child-like personality, as so many of us do when we grow up. To him, anything was possible. This type of existence granted him more creativity, adventure, and spontaneity. Doesn't that sound inviting? I, too, want to have a carefree attitude like his.

The course also discussed the need for self-care. If we want to be of better service to others, we need to nourish ourselves. In class, we were taught additional ways to work on self-care – to meditate and go in with a child's curiosity – wielding no expectations and having fun. Acknowledge that the child within may have past hurts and may still be wounded – sometimes our relationship with our more vulnerable selves must be rekindled. As the saying goes, "Feelings buried never die." I have further developed self-trust and am transforming my life one step at a time through my personal experiences. I left class that day feeling more excited than ever.

FOCUSING ON SELF-LOVE

A mind that is stretched by a new experience
can never go back to its old dimensions.

~ Oliver Wendell Holmes

It's October 13, 2020, and I had another appointment with my herbalist, whom I see every three to four months. At the end of our session, he told me that my body was in a reset mode. I asked if that was a good thing, and his response was optimistic. He made a few adjustments to my current herbal tincture (as he often does) to help with my body's transition. I left with excitement, ready to confidently take on life's unknowns and face the new day. I am the seed of my power and have the ability to nourish it to fruition. With this in mind, I was looking forward to the upcoming Healing Touch course and prepared myself to indulge even further in my child-like curiosity. After this fourth class, I will only need to pass one more level before becoming a certified Healing Touch Practitioner. Of course, there is additional required coursework to complete for certification, but I am almost there!

When course four began in this same month of October, we chose a partner with which we would exchange eight sessions. Over the next few days, my partner and I split up our roles so that we would each be the practitioner for four of the sessions and the client for the other four. Both practitioner and client experiences were memorable, but serving as a client felt the most profound. My first client session began as usual with my eyes closed, and I laid in a relaxed state on the massage table. During the session, I had another vision of a lion, a hawk, and the top of a shoe. Next, my grandma appeared, and we visited. Memories flowed through my mind, and I relived snippets of our time together. It was surreal.

My second session as a client was a bit more dramatic. My practitioner partner was working with me, and, from the sound of her discreet sniffles, I sensed that she was crying. Instead of interfering, I decided to keep my eyes closed and continued focusing on the mental image coming into view. Like Tinker Bell in the *Peter Pan* story, I saw myself as a fairy. Only, it was *my* face with a tiny pixie-like body and wings, just like Tinker Bell's. I was happily flying over my body (as I laid on the massage table) and pulling out the things that no longer served me. Suddenly, I grasped onto something much heavier. I needed to use all of my might to hoist a large, black briefcase out of my core area. I pulled as hard as I could, and my fairy dust started flying in all directions. Finally, the briefcase gave way, and I threw it so far that it could no longer be seen with the eye. When my session was over, I felt much lighter. It was as if nothing was holding me back.

However, when I looked at my partner to see if she felt similarly, she had a grave, shaken-up expression on her face. She told me that nothing like this had happened while she was giving a Healing Touch treatment before. When she was working with me, she had felt so much sadness. In fact, it was an overwhelming amount. The deep-rooted feeling had made her cry. She asked me if I was really sick while going through my treatments. I said, "Yes, why do you ask? Would you like more information from me?" She nodded, and I knew that something of great significance had just occurred.

I told her that at one point, I went into the spirit world and chose to come back for my children – a 'breath of life' made this possible. My partner started to cry and said, "I saw you on the hospital bed. Only, you were gray in color, cold to the touch, and had no life in you. Your physical body was dead. But then, you took a deep breath and slowly came back to life, like 'new' – all the illness was gone. Your cheeks became flushed and rosy, and your arms were in a different position. You were still in the hospital bed, but your eyes were open, and you were alive." She went on to say, "During our session, there were so many good people around you, like an entourage, watching over you." We both sobbed as I told her about my vision of being a fairy and joyfully releasing the things that no longer served me in a child-like way. It was as if I was clearing out the dead to make room for more love and light, like every bit of residual pain was GONE, forever. Our exchange of energy made one message exceptionally clear...

I am healed.

 James 1:2-4 ~ Consider it pure joy, my brothers and sisters, whenever you face trials of many kinds, because you know that the testing of your faith produces perseverance. Let perseverance finish its work so that you may be mature and complete, not lacking anything.

ROOM TO FLOURISH

 Psalm 30:2 ~ LORD my God, I called to you for help, and you healed me.

CURED. Now that's a word that causes spiritual goosebumps to appear across my entire body. What an extraordinary feeling it holds.

I still think about the breath of life that my Lord so graciously gifted me during my first experience with cancer. And for the longest time, I questioned why my illness returned in May of 2017. How could it be possible when I had a BREATH OF LIFE? Wasn't this second chance supposed to be the BIG sign that my trial was over? For lack of a better phrase, my relapse was a slap in the face. I did everything the medical care team told me to do for long-term remission and a cure. So, why *me*?

I took a step back and reflected, "Did I *really* do everything?" It seemed like I had healed and fallen right back into my former toxic habits. I also feel that I allowed my fears of leukemia to replay in my mind. Deep within, there was still a speck of anxiety every time I heard the word cancer, triggering an unrelenting sensation in the pit of my stomach. I hadn't learned everything that I needed to from my first experience, so God felt it was necessary to put me through leukemia one more time. My ultimate closure opened doors I didn't even know were there, including those of universal energy through the modalities of Reiki, Herbalist Program, and more recently, Healing Touch.

These new opportunities get me thinking about how we spend our time. How do we know what to prioritize? Suppose we put a price tag on time and treat it as any other grocery store necessity. Does the relationship between supply and demand hold true? Think about it. Do your minutes become more valuable once they start ticking down to the last few intervals? And when time is stolen from you, as years of my life were ripped away by cancer, don't you feel completely defeated? Time is something that we often don't consider until our space is interrupted by unwanted obstacles.

After meditating on time for a while, I've realized how much our society takes our freedom for granted. We all seem to have a 'GO-GO-GO' mentality, driven by work, school, and other responsibilities. Trust me, I understand that it's difficult to hit the pause button, but after missing out on so much during my hospital stays, I know that slowing down is imperative. Time is the one thing in life that we can never get back. We ought to be spending it how we want to.

Reflecting back further, I wish I had taken more time for myself even before cancer. My virulent impulses to put everyone else first made me miss out on my interests and joys. As I said before, I suppose a bit of struggle is okay since it brought me to my current state of enlightenment. Now, when I notice the beginning stages of frustration and anxiety, I try to rid myself of whatever is compromising my efficiency. I'm not suggesting that you quit your job or abandon your family, but rather that you think more about YOUR purpose, YOUR goals, and YOUR values. Consider if your current obligations define your true self. And if they aren't measuring up, reevaluate your schedule to make time for the activities you love most.

Here is a list of healthy practices that ease the mind and maximize our time:

- Exercise – any type of movement. It could be cardio, yoga, pilates, or a brisk walk with your dog.
- Reorganize drawers or storage areas in your house and purge the unwanted items. It always makes me feel good when I have a tidy living space.
- Try a new recipe. Perhaps it will become a new favorite!

- Check out Pinterest for craft or art ideas. Get inspired!

- Watch a romantic comedy from Hallmark with a glass of wine. Maybe bring along a tub of ice cream for good measure.

- Go somewhere by yourself to recharge. It could be a nature hike, a coffee shop indulgence, or even a trip to the store.

- Meditate or empty your thoughts through a guided deep-relaxation soundtrack. Sometimes I bring a notebook and pen if I am inspired to write about whatever moves me or needs released. Sometimes burning what you write provides the greatest relief.

- Practice deep-breathing techniques, and focus on nothing but your inhales and exhales for a few minutes.

- Drink a warm cup of tea and read a book in a quiet space.

- Listen to soothing music, or make some music yourself. Playing an instrument and singing is an outlet like no other.

- Take a relaxing candle-lit bath with added aromas of Epsom salt and essential oils.

- Spend quality time with family. Did somebody say GAME NIGHT?!

- Take a nap. You may be working yourself way too hard. Listen to your body.

- Go on vacation! Spend time in an exotic location to improve awareness. Explore the tropics, the historical sites, or the mountains. The world has so much to offer.

- Go on an outing with friends. Reconnect and reminisce on the joys of the past while also taking time to make new memories.

- Phone a relative or an old friend to get some words of encouragement. You'd be surprised by the number of people who care to listen.

- Do something nice for someone to lift both your spirit *and* theirs.

- Take time to learn something new, like playing the guitar or crocheting.

- Join an online book club or get a new book from the library. Develop a bond with like-minded people.

The list goes on and on. These are just some of my go-to ideas. How you delegate your free time will determine your level of fulfillment. My advice is not to waste too many hours on material matters. There is so much love surrounding you, like family, friends, pets, hobbies, and nature. If we don't look up, we'll get stuck in a perpetual rift of unhappiness. Allow me to elaborate:

The universe is full of patterns... so much so that their presence has become inevitable; repetitions weave their way into nature, mathematics, and, most often, our social lives. Even with this systematic connection, however, it's challenging to recognize the roles patterns play in our lives. Consistent experiences sprout questions like, "Why does this particular scenario keep replaying in my life? Is this recurrence improving my outlook? What steps can I take to overcome my habit with ease?"

Let's face it, we all prefer to walk through life with security, and sometimes it's easiest just to accept the uncomfortable; the downside of this preference is that our goals will become fogged over. For example, I've begun to realize I'm terrified of negative responses, and as a result, I play things too safe. Over time, as my desires are sacrificed for the contentment of others, my unmet needs spiral into dissatisfaction. And it doesn't end there. The discontent helixes collide and expand into 'safety nets of familiarity' that trap us as much as they protect us. This underlying cycle eats away at our identity until we are forced to shift our attitude into a more grounded state.

Unfortunately, abandoning the built-up facades is anything but easy. All sorts of obstacles will stand in our way. It is only once we are able to make it past the inconveniences that the clarity of our purpose will shine through.

Looking deeper into the hardships of conformity, does it ever feel like everyone is fundamentally facing the same trials repeatedly? Do politics, arguments, and misunderstandings ever start to blur together? When I examine our population, why is a collection of messes the only thing I see? As Albert Einstein says, "We cannot solve our problems with the same thinking we used when we created them." We need to take a moment to break out of our habits and recalibrate.

Einstein's quote is relevant in *all* of life's challenges and oddly reminds me of my battle with CANcer; my illness repeated itself because I wasn't introduced to everything I was destined to learn after the first occurrence.

Perhaps my pattern of CANcer manifested because I had fallen back into those unwanted routines. I needed an impetus to snap me out of it.

Upon this discovery, I finally understood what my soul's progression required. The first step in branching out of my comfort zone was resigning from my teaching position. Although I knew in my heart that I needed to quit for some time, I let the expectations of others and the fear of consequences control my actions. I was worried about how my family would be affected and how my colleagues would react. Most of all, I didn't want my legacy, specifically with the Sensory Courtyard where "Seeds Sown Today Bring Blossoms Tomorrow," to be forgotten or deemed useless. These anxieties fueled my indecisiveness and reinforced my patterns of isolation and friction. None of my puzzle pieces were fitting together, no matter how hard I shoved them into the picture. This collective build-up of emotions was challenging to overcome, but for the first time in a while, I felt ready to blindly bargain on new opportunities.

Battles of the heart and mind will always be there, but I can assure you that each step towards authenticity makes the pressures easier to overcome. And don't worry about the footprints you leave behind! Memories and relations will fade, but your journey is eternal. It's time to give up the illusion of control and invite divine wellness.

With that being said, what is my final destination in this lifetime? Will I be reunited with the special souls who helped mark my path? Will they bop me on my head for missing prime opportunities in my faith journey? These rapid questions made another realization become all the more clear – without the companionship of others, humans are left with only the echoes of themselves.

Although we are most honest with ourselves in solitude, the most dynamic form of growth stems from relationships. Influence from outsiders has the potential to both provide insight and lead us astray. But, as I made clear in the beginning of this story, sometimes the most painful interactions inspire the grandest of transformations.

The two-time CANcer journey was the most difficult trial I've ever gone through, and I couldn't imagine going through it alone. Life is much easier now that things are calm and still, but during times of trouble, it's beneficial to keep this well-known quote in mind: The greater your storm, the brighter your rainbow.

There is another lesson here: The storms help us find our weaknesses and give us insight into changes we need to make. God targets us with disturbances to help us make discoveries about ourselves. James 1:2-4 states, "Consider it pure joy, my brothers and sisters, whenever you face trials of many kinds, because you know that the testing of your faith produces perseverance. Let perseverance finish its work so that you may be mature and complete, not lacking anything." As we persevere through emotional states of disorder and finish the race God has marked out for us, I believe we will be welcomed into the afterlife with these comforting words: "Well done, good, and faithful servant."

When I'm asked about my current passion, the answer is simple – Universal energy. I love to help others by tapping into the light of the universe and offering support. And it's crazy to think that I would never have discovered natural healing without the stepping stone of cancer. I am so happy that Reiki and Healing Touch led me to a newfound state of contentment.

As for any connection with my stem cell transplant donor? After receiving no responses from three separate occasions of sending him emails, I had accepted it as a lost cause. However, on August 24, 2021, I was thrilled to see that he had finally gotten back to me! My donor wrote that he hadn't received my first or second emails because they must have gone to the spam filter. Thank goodness I never gave up! I'm also glad that I sent the emails to Stephan on the same email thread so he could read everything my family and I had written to him since May 2020.

As a final thought, I would like to reflect on my journey as a whole. God planted the seed of my destiny the moment I was born, but my uncertainties and suppressions prevented its growth. Sometimes weeds refuse to leave, and there's no other solution than to spray them with poison. My CANcer was brutal, but my stem held firm with the help of the stem cell transplant and continued growing through the heat of the drought. Eventually, the rain and sun came back, and there were no longer any weeds holding me back. My plant was finally able to bloom in the way that God had intended all along. The extermination of burdens has given me so much more room to flourish. It's only up from here!

 Psalm 9:1 ~ I will give thanks to you, LORD, with all my heart; I will tell of all your wonderful deeds.

ACKNOWLEDGMENTS

I would like to thank:

God, my rock, my redeemer, my EVERYTHING. I am grateful for every day You have given me on Earth and intend to make every moment count. Thank You for steering the wheel (especially when I was unable to myself) and driving me toward the discovery of natural healing. Universal energy is an outlet that's improved both my confidence and strengths – especially those of my courage and character. It's humbling to share Your wonders with others. My life is Yours alone.

Heather Doyle Fraser with the Compassionate Mind Collaborative for helping my book come to fruition with your knowledge and expertise regarding the mechanics of book-writing. *Seed, Stem, Bloom* would not be what it is today without your support and guidance. You are an invaluable coach, providing attention to detail, insight, and a collaborative mind. Thank you for believing in my writing abilities and my story. You will forever hold a special place in my heart. Sending you love, light, and immense gratitude.

To my production team at the Compassionate Mind Collaborative: Dino Marino, thank you for bringing my words to life with your lovely designs and creative genius. Your flexibility and willingness to satisfy my vision mean the world to me. Jesse Sussman, your marketing guidance has been incredibly helpful in my book's premiere. I honestly don't know what I would have done without you. And Julie Homon, thank you for your attention to detail in the final proofing of the book. Each conclusive tweak makes an extreme difference, and I hope it's clear how much I appreciate all three of you.

My husband, Tim, for keeping my spirits up, even on the darkest days. You have a beautiful gift of generating laughter. Your silly jokes somehow continue to be funny even though I've heard them over and over. I'm also grateful for your ability to find joy in any experience. Thank you for taking the bad with the good and never giving up on me. You are more than

I could ever ask for in a partner, and I'm blessed to have such a loving companion and best friend.

My children – Brody, Holly, Colby, and Shaylee – for the unconditional love, support, and encouragement when I needed it most. I am incredibly proud of the person each of you has become and look forward to witnessing your bright futures blossom on your journey. I love you with all that I am, and then some! You are my light; thank you for inspiring me to be a better person.

A special thanks to my daughter, Holly, for always being there when I have writer's block and need to find a better way to share my thoughts on paper. Somehow, you find a way to make any sentence or paragraph magnificent. You are so talented and successful at anything you set your mind to accomplish. Don't ever lose sight of your dreams! You have so many gifts to offer this world and have already made a significant impact on the lives of others with your compassionate heart. Always let your light shine brightly.

A special thanks to my son, Brody, who – at the young age of sixteen – didn't hesitate to go through various blood withdrawals to find out if he was the best stem cell match to save my life. You are so giving, optimistic, and willing to go the extra mile to help loved ones. We are very fortunate that your younger siblings have such a great role model.

My parents, Ernie and Jane Hall: You have guided and shaped me into the woman I am today. I have been blessed with the two most selfless, kind-hearted parents, and I can't thank you enough for being who you are. You demonstrate good Christian morals and values daily and continue to lend a hand whenever the family needs it. Thank you for encouraging me to follow my passions and for always believing in me. I strive to be like you – my heroes.

My brother, Matt, who has always been someone I've looked up to. I couldn't have asked for a better sibling. You do whatever it takes to help me in any situation – especially in the case of potentially being my stem cell transplant match. Your witty sense of humor and positive spin on challenges always have a way of lifting my spirits. Thank you for being there for me, even when hundreds of miles separate us. Your encouragement has made me believe that I can do anything I set my mind to, including writing this book.

My mother-in-law, Vickie, who consistently showers me with love. You have welcomed me into your side of the family from day one, and I am grateful for such a supportive extension of relatives. Additionally, thank you for all the crocheted items you've gifted me over the years. Each unique design holds value and loving memories. I am especially grateful for the vibrant striped crocheted blanket you gave me while in the hospital. Each color represents the birthstone of my family members. This specially-designed blanket provided a feeling of peace and love in a time when I needed it most.

Thank you to all of the doctors, nurses, caregivers, chaplains, and medical professionals who helped me on my road to recovery at Methodist Hospital, Methodist Estabrook Cancer Center, Nebraska Medicine, and Fred & Pamela Buffett Cancer Center. Specifically, Dr. Timothy Huyck, oncologist at Nebraska Cancer Specialists; Dr. Vijaya Bhatt, oncologist at Nebraska Medicine; and Nicholas Schnell, Clinical Herbalist, RH, LMNT at Four Winds Natural Healing Center. Thank you to all the individuals who work in the medical field to help others. You make a difference!

To countless friends, colleagues, extended family, churches, and the general public, I am beyond grateful for your prayers, acts of kindness, and support – especially in my desperate time of need. You are a testament to the power of LOVE. Your encouragement on my original CaringBridge site started it all, and I'm not sure if I would have had the courage to write this book without your influence. Thank you for the many blessings. Sending love to all.

ABOUT THE AUTHOR

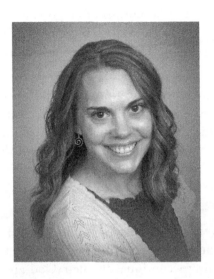

Mary Jane Robinson is a warrior.

She is a mom, wife, sister, daughter, teacher, and healer. Mary is determined – accustomed to putting on the Armor of God and going to battle.

After not feeling well in 2014, this always-on-the-go woman had a diagnosis that not only changed her perspective on life but also deepened her commitment to the one she already had. A bone marrow biopsy confirmed that Mary had acute myeloid leukemia (AML). A relapse in 2017 determined that an allogeneic stem cell transplant was the only option for long-term survival. During her fight for life, Mary was introduced to Reiki – a Japanese form of energy healing – and eventually became a Reiki Master/Teacher. From there, she began learning about Healing Touch, which is another energy healing modality involving therapeutic touch. In 2018, Mary completed a two-year program through Prairie Star Center for Herbal Studies and became a certified herbalist. In the fall of 2020, Mary was named an ordained minister through the Universal Brotherhood Movement, Inc.

Mary's husband, Tim, owns a land surveying business called American Surveyors, Inc., and they have four children – Brody, Holly, Colby, and Shaylee. They reside on acreage in the country and enjoy many outdoor activities. One of their favorite places to relax is the family cabin that rests along the Platte River. The Robinsons often go kayaking, floating, airboat riding, and walking in nature. Mary's indoor activities include reading, writing, cooking, organizing, and watching a good film with her family.

Prior to her cancer diagnosis in 2014, Mary earned Bachelor of Science endorsements in elementary education and mild to moderate disabilities through Chadron State College in 2001. She went on to earn a Master of Arts in special education, with an emphasis in visual impairments, through the University of Nebraska – Lincoln in 2009. And she didn't stop there! In 2011, Mary achieved an orientation and mobility endorsement through the University of Northern Colorado, becoming certified in orientation and mobility in 2012.

It has always been one of Mary's passions to work with students of special needs. She finds it very rewarding to help others reach new heights and teach them skills to continue on their God-given journey. During the majority of her career, Mary was a teacher of the visually impaired and provided orientation and mobility services to students from birth through twenty-one years of age. Mary was one of sixteen teachers chosen nationwide to be in the first Teacher of Tomorrow Program of 2010-2011. This program, hosted by the National Federation of the Blind, helped establish a network system with other teachers and leaders in the visually impaired community. These connections better equipped Mary to prepare her students for the real world.

In addition to these singular accomplishments, Mary is also the founder of the Sensory Courtyard, where "Seeds Sown Today Bring Blossoms Tomorrow." The Sensory Courtyard covers approximately three thousand square feet and is located in Fremont, Nebraska. This interactive space consists of specialized educational areas, each designed to spark the senses in a different way.

Mary's story gives hope and reassurance. Her perseverance confirms the power of a positive mindset and faith.

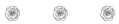

If readers are interested in being on the donation list for stem cells, they can go to www.BetheMatch.org website to register. Be the Match will send a swab kit for potential donors to swab inside their mouth (cheek) and return. They will be added to the general population pool. Every life is precious and any donor could be the match for someone and save a life.

If readers are interested in donating blood, contact your local Red Cross or your community blood center to verify your eligibility and help save lives.

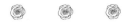

Made in the USA
Middletown, DE
11 April 2022

63915635R00163